For Rachel

I

Infertility Insanity

Infertility Insanity

When sheer hope (and Google)
are the only options left

Julie Selby

First Published in Canada 2015 by Influence Publishing

Book Cover Design: Patrick John Aldana
Editing Team: Nina Shoroplova and Jennifer Kaleta
Typeset: Greg Salisbury
Photographer: Luiza Matysiak

Library and Archives Canada Cataloguing in Publication

Selby, Julie, 1968-, author
    Infertility insanity : when sheer hope (and Google)
are the only options left / Julie Selby.

ISBN 978-1-77141-024-3 (pbk.)

1. Selby, Julie, 1968-. 2. Infertility. I. Title.

RG201.S45 2014   618.1'78   C2014-904806-8

Testimonials

"As a Family Therapist I understand that the topic of infertility is emotional and often difficult to discuss. Julie Selby takes a different approach in talking about her experiences. Her compelling story, laced with humour, takes a uniquely honest look at the struggles with infertility that so many women and couples face."
Alyson Jones, President of Alyson Jones and Associates, Child and Family Therapist, Author of "MORE: A New Philosophy for Exceptional Living"

"Infertility Insanity is a heartfelt and humorous account of one woman's journey from 'unfertile' to 'fertile.' Filled with raw honesty and lively descriptions of real people with real fertility issues, this book will make you laugh, cry and cheer for Julie and Sam. This is a must-read for anyone grappling with the intensity of infertility."
Lisa Martin, Leadership Coach, Bestselling Author of "Briefcase Moms"

"Julie Selby has written a book on infertility unlike any other. Infertility Insanity offers a deeply personal look into the author's journey to get pregnant and so much more. Infused with warmth, humour, tears and hope, Selby opens a window into a world that will keep you riveted from start to finish."
Marilyn R. Wilson, Editor, Raine Magazine

"Infertility is an emotional rollercoaster, and at times can leave you feeling completely overwhelmed and isolated. Reading about other experiences, such as Julie's frank and honest account of her journey, can help you understand that you are not mad, bad, or completely insane, and that others too feel the same as you!"
Susan Seenan, Chief Executive, Infertility Network UK

Acknowledgements

This book was on my mind for seven years and probably would have stayed there without the help and support of an amazing group of family and friends.

There was "Sam," who didn't bat an eyelid when I left my well-paying job to finally get this story down on paper. He was the first one to read the manuscript and urge me to share it with the world—his main edit being correcting (up) his sperm count numbers! His support, trust and encouragement never wavered, even when the bills started piling up. Thanks, Sam.

To my incredible bunch of girlfriends, who pushed me along the way, thank you for supplying me with wine and encouragement when I had second thoughts. You're a tough bunch of cookies, but I wouldn't want to be without you all for a second.

Thank you to Sam's and my families for the support both emotionally and financially, especially my Mum and my sister who, although they're living halfway around the world, never once questioned what I was doing and had complete faith that I would finish this book one day. Apologies to Mum, who after reading it said, "Well, I think I know more about your sex life now than I ever needed to!"

To the team at Influence Publishing, thank you for helping me find my path through this story and for challenging me to do my best. Special gratitude to Nina and Julie whose patience and editing helped me take my story to the next level.

I couldn't close this without acknowledging the fertility team at the clinic. You change people's lives every day. A big thank you to "Dr. T.," who was patient, wise, funny and who gave me two remarkable, spirited, and precious little beings.

Thank you.

Contents

Dedication...I

Testimonials.. III

Acknowledgements V

Preface... IX

Tick. Tock. Tick. Tock.. 1

Misery Loves Company 19

The Point of No Return.. 35

Talking to the Dead 55

Insanity Starts to Take Over.. 63

Go Big or Go Home... 93

Art and Love.. 111

The Last Kick at the Can... 119

Make or Break... 133

The Home Stretch... 155

Epilogue 169

Author Biography 173

Preface

If you are going through infertility and have found this book, you are probably either online or in a bookstore trying to find something, anything, that will help you get pregnant, or perhaps you know someone who is struggling with infertility and want to help. Or finally, you are my Mum, who promised me that she would buy at least five copies.

During my five-year infertility journey, I lost count of how many hours I spent in bookstores and online trying to find the answers for my diagnosis of "unexplained infertility." There are some great books and information sources out there on infertility; most are written from a medical or "how to get pregnant" perspective, but I was looking for the one that would guarantee me a baby or at least that I could relate to when I felt like I was losing my mind. I needed something that would offer ideas I hadn't tried yet or just light relief in the dark days. By the way, there are none that guarantee you a baby, and I didn't find too many of the other ones either, which was the impetus for this one.

This story is mainly my story. It is about how infertility can literally make you lose your mind, how it impacts every aspect of your life, how hope is the only thing that keeps you going, and how, when you don't have an answer, you are prepared to try anything (by "anything," I mean "anything," including past life regression, art therapy and talking to dead people).

But this story is also about my friends. There is Maxine, who was dealing with infertility then had to take on cancer; my sister, who was diagnosed with PCOS and had her own infertility journey; and Kari who, after a ten-year quest for her own children, found an alternate route. However, if you are going through infertility and do not want to hear yet another story with a happy ending, you should stop here. I totally get it. I was one of the lucky ones.

The world of infertility (or as I have now re-named it,

"unfertility," for reasons explained in the book) is not a fun place. It is miserable and I wish someone had prepared me for it. I had no idea how dark and, at times, bizarre this world would be. For me, trying to find some humour in the situations I found myself in helped me cope. I hope it helps you too.

Good luck.

Julie Selby

Tick. Tock. Tick. Tock.

I can't quite remember exactly when we started trying for a baby "naturally." My best guess is just after my thirty-fifth birthday. Sam was keen to get going, but in truth I was not quite as enthusiastic. I was loving my job and my life, hence the "starting age" of thirty-five. We did what we wanted, we had no responsibilities, and there was a nagging thought at the back of my mind that maybe I wouldn't be a great mother. This was rooted in issues from my past. I have seen how perfectly normal parents can really (unintentionally) screw up their children.

Here's a little bit of my history. I grew up in a small town in Lincolnshire, England, called Bourne. I have one sister called Jane who is three years older than me. My Mum and Dad were both working class, we lived in a semi-detached, we holidayed in England, we grocery-shopped on Fridays, had fish and chips occasionally, probably watched a bit too much TV (but "colour" was new then), had several dogs that died, and a ferret that tried to eat my eyeball once. Overall, I would say a pretty normal child-hood. My parents worked very hard to make sure we did not go without. They had not had the privilege of a good education themselves, so they made sure we worked hard at school. They also loved each other, a lot.

Education for me was a way to both return the favour to my Mum and Dad, and also to escape Bourne. When you are fifteen and living in a town that has ten pubs, most within fifty feet of each other, and very little else, you do start to wonder what the outside world is like. The only industry in the town at the time was agriculture and by the time I was sixteen, I had worked at a variety of jobs, the highlights being pea grader, cauliflower breaker-upper, strawberry picker, vegetable chopper, and, my favourite random one, maker of fibreglass arms for plastic robots. My sister also figured out that she needed to explore the world. Her strategy was to leave at seventeen, as she had met her Prince Charming who lived somewhere else and was ready to whisk her away. I had no Prince Charming and no such escape plan, so the only way for me to leave was to go to university; I chose Newcastle University in North East England. Funny, now when I go back, I think what a great place Bourne was to grow up in. My Mum has never forgiven either of us for leaving and not staying close by, but, as I pointed out, it was she and Dad who kept saying, "Explore the world." So be careful what you tell your kids.

I originally came to Vancouver because of my ex-boyfriend Adam. We had been seeing each other on and off since university and it was one of those intense relationships. Post-university I moved to London and Adam went to Leeds in the UK. Being part of Generation X, timing has never been my strong point and when I graduated it was a time of recession. So this meant going where the jobs were. And for me that was London. I was sad Adam and I would not be together, but I was also excited. I had never lived in London, and, coming from a small town, "London" sounded very grown up and cosmopolitan. I even caught myself one day saying I was moving to "The Smoke." I think I had heard the term used on TV and thought I would sound like a native Londoner. I didn't. I sounded like an idiot.

Long story short. Adam got an opportunity to move to Vancouver and I had twenty-four hours to make up my mind about whether I was going to go with him. I went to bed that night, thought I had nothing to lose, and agreed. Adam left six months before me. In the time he was away, I moved jobs, applied for my landed immigrant visa, took some French lessons, as you got more points on the application form for that, and basically life went on as normal.

As my leaving date drew closer though, I began phoning Adam at odd times of the day and night. Something felt wrong. Well, it was in fact very wrong. About a week before I was due to fly out, he called. He wanted to let me know that he had met someone else and wasn't sure it was such a good idea for me to come. No bloody kidding! I had given up my job, my flat, and was packed and ready to leave to start a new life with someone I thought was, on the whole, a pretty decent guy.

I put the phone down and called my friend Sue. To this day I will never forget what she did. She got in her car, drove a couple of hundred miles that night, arrived with a bottle of gin, and stayed up with me all night as I blubbered and drank myself into oblivion. The next day, she got up at some god-unearthly hour and drove back to work. That is a rare friend.

But now I had to decide what to do. Part of me just wanted to stick my head under the pillow and forget the whole Vancouver thing, but I couldn't, even though that would have been the mature thing to do. I decided that, despite being dramatically dumped and usurped by some no-doubt perfect-toothed West Coast individual who spent her days rollerblading, this was not going to deter me from getting on that plane.

My parents and friends thought I was bonkers. I had never been to Vancouver, was heartbroken, at this point hung over most of the time, had no place to stay, and knew no one there. But what they didn't factor in was that I had told everyone I was going. It was purely my ego that forced me on that plane. That and the fact that, after dating Adam for seven years, I thought he and I should at least meet face-to-face. I told him I was coming, and could actually feel him blanche through the phone line. Sitting on the plane, I suddenly realized what I had done; I felt it was probably one of my stupidest moves to date.

There is a much longer story that continues after this, but for the purpose of this book, the scenario was as follows. Arrived in Vancouver. Lived with Adam for a week. Had some great break-up sex. Moved out and decided that if I could get a job in six weeks, I would stay. But I swore off any kind of relationship for at least eighteen months, so I could heal or do whatever you are meant to do after being unceremoniously dumped for, as I later found out, a younger model. The good news is Adam is a good guy, we are still in touch, and time (along with alcohol) really does heal all things.

I got a job within six weeks, answered an ad for a house share, and started to set up my new life. With a new job, a good flat mate, and a gradual understanding of how the West Coast of Canada operates, I began to find my pioneering spirit.

One of the things I found most difficult was making friends. I have heard many people say this over the seventeen years I have lived here, but Vancouver was, certainly at that time anyway, very cliquey. Very rarely did people invite you into their group of friends. I remember so many conversations where people would casually say, "We should go for a drink" and I would reply like an eager puppy, "Great, when? I'm pretty free most evenings from now until the rest of the year," and they would run for the door!

Work was not much easier. There were some great people where I worked but, unlike in the UK where everyone goes for a drink after work and usually ends up making a spectacular career-limiting move by drinking too much, here it seemed people went jogging, rollerblading, or mountain climbing. None of which really appealed to me, but hey, when in Rome.

The first thing I did was buy some new workout gear. I noticed everyone was not only thin, but stylishly thin. The second thing I did was join a volleyball team. My team was made up of Aussies, New Zealanders, and Brits, none of whom could actually play and all of whom had only signed up to meet other people. I think we had one Canadian who left fairly quickly after seeing the level of our expertise.

One day we were short a player and that was the day Sam arrived.

Sam is also a Brit, but, uncharacteristically for our team, he knew how to play volleyball and was competitive. This was a whole new concept to us and one that did not go down well. Within minutes of Sam arriving and seeing the desperate state of our skills, he quickly became frustrated and started yelling at us. Now normally I would think, "What a dick," but for some reason I was distracted by the fact that he had lovely thighs and wore his T-shirt very well. By the end of the game, he was ready to throw in the towel, said he would never play with such a lame team again, and I was quite certain that I was going to be in a long-term relationship with him. I was particularly annoyed as I had promised myself that I would not date anyone for eighteen months and this was only a year into the eighteen months. That said, I told myself, the universe, and whoever else was listening, that if he bothered to find out my number then I would have to date him.

Three weeks later, I was away on business filming in Toronto when I checked my voicemail and there was a message from Sam. He was wondering if I wanted to go for a drink when I was back in Vancouver. Shit! Now, I would have to go.

I remember that first date. It went quite well considering I was thinking of bailing just beforehand. That was until Sam said that he had attended Newcastle University. I was very curious as that was also my university, and I knew a lot of people there—Sam was not one of them. I had graduated in 1988. It was now 1997. And I was 28.

I asked Sam when he had graduated.

He replied, "This year."

"Bloody hell," I said, "How old are you?"

"Twenty three," he said.

Oh God! I went home thinking this could not possibly work; Sam went home, called his Mum, and said, "I think I have met the next Mrs. Dexter."

Throughout my life, I have had an issue with relationships and commitment. I actually had doubts that I was capable of sustaining a relationship and unequivocally committing to one person for life. I so admire those couples who meet and just know he or she is "the one." How does that happen? I have spoken to a lot of people about this and they say that yes, for some people, it is a bolt of lightning and they have complete clarity about the "rightness" of their partner. However, I have also spoken to just as many who have said that it's a matter of "committing" and "choosing."

For me with Sam, it was a combination of the two. When I saw him, I knew I was in for the long haul, but I also "chose" him. Ideally, given the choice, I would have liked to have been struck by a lightning bolt. It just feels more romantic. Plus Holy Moly ... if you make the choice ... then it is completely your fault if it goes tits-up, and you can't blame a random thunderbolt from the heavens.

And ultimately, let's face it, in all likelihood there are probably a number of people in this world who you could be extremely happy with. I find it incredible that with six billion people on earth, you can find your soul mate in the house next door, or the village you grew up in, or, in my case, on a volleyball court in Vancouver.

Thus we began our relationship. It started off slowly as I think we were both cautious. Me, because of my past experiences, and Sam, because he just likes to take his time. In all my time of knowing Sam, I have never seen him rush. Even if he is worried about being late and will say, miss the bus, he still will not run. Hurrying is just not in his DNA. His Mum once told me a story about how when he was younger, even when he was really late for school, he would not eat his cereal any faster. His Mum got so frustrated that, in the end, she just picked up the cereal bowl and dumped the contents on his head. The irony was that Sam wouldn't leave until he had had some more cereal.

We dated for about two years and then decided we would move in together. The night before the move, I remember being in complete angst. Not because I didn't think it was a good idea, but I had never lived with anyone and was panicking about how it would go.

Surprisingly, it was good. We soon figured out that we were opposites when it came to co-habiting. Me ... messy, but clean. Sam ... anally tidy, but not necessarily clean. When I left the kitchen after making dinner, it looked like a food slaughter had taken place. The food was good, the clean-up job was big. Sam was usually on clean-up and I noticed over time that he kept offering to make dinner, just because he couldn't face the kitchen afterwards. This would have been great, but Sam's idea of a sauce was usually a blob of ketchup and some grated cheese.

We still continually work on balancing our habits. It will never be perfect, but I am tidier and Sam now adds real tomatoes to his sauces.

We had a lot of fun. We travelled, made lots of good friends, and had some good adventures. We both enjoyed our jobs. Sam was in construction management and I worked with an advertising agency that I loved. We talked about children, but not very seriously. I was "on the fence" at the time. Sam was definitely in the "kids camp." After we had been together for about four years, he wanted to know when I would be ready to have a baby. My reply was always, "Not yet." But one thing about Sam is he is very determined and when he puts his mind to something, he can be relentless.

After buying an apartment, being together for seven years, and approaching the biological clock "death zone" of being thirty-five years old, the "not yet" reply was not cutting it. Sam was getting impatient and I realized that if I was going to live a life of no regrets (my current philosophy of the time; I have had a few philosophies, the most disastrous of which was "Eat and be happy," and I am still dealing with the consequences of that one!), then I had to get off the fence and get on with it or I was going to lose Sam. And I didn't want that.

Sam is one of the few guys who can make me laugh. His most famous line during one of our "baby discussions" was, "Look Ju, you are not getting any younger; things will start to drop and droop soon; I may be your best and last chance!" I know most women would have a fit, but for some reason his delivery always made me smile and I knew he loved me. So, after another of these discussions, we agreed. It was time. I mean, God forbid that I would be left a drooping, sagging mess of loneliness on the shelf!

So I committed and got working on the job of procreation. At first, because you think you will get pregnant straight away, it's good sex. You do it because it's fun and because you now don't have to worry about protection. You don't really watch which days you are having sex, since, hey, you are just enjoying the training. This lasts for a few months. Then you realize that okay, maybe getting pregnant is not as easy as you thought. You suddenly start thinking that you should "plan" your sex a little more. You are officially entering Stage One of "trying" for a baby.

This stage is what I think of as "education and the warm-up." In the case of many women, it seems they are in tune with their body when ovulating. Not so for me. When I engaged the services of my best friend, Google, I was quite shocked that I had made it to thirty-five without really having a clue about how my own reproductive system works. I knew the basics: periods, ovulation about halfway between periods. But, after getting online, I realized I was a complete novice. Women on forums were talking about basal body temperatures (BBTs), viscosity of discharge and fluid, and egg eruption. I must admit, I felt a bit freaked out. There was something frantic about the exchanges on the forums. Reading women's discussions about the "stickiness" of the fluid leaving their most private parts was definitely out of my comfort zone.

However, basal temperatures made sense as I learned that Stage One is really about figuring out when you ovulate, as you can conceive one or two days on either side of this. Off to the pharmacy I went. This was when I experienced my first real sense of the importance I would be placing on every decision in the baby-making process. There must have been about five brands of basal temperature measuring devices, from some big brand names to the store's own brand.

I asked for help in deciding which one to buy. Basically, I was told they all did about the same kind of job, some more sophisticatedly than others. Arghhh! I suddenly panicked a bit, I started obsessing over which stupid one to buy as I wanted to make sure I chose the "right" one. The one that would help me get a baby. I asked so many questions about reliability, reviews, etc., that eventually the lovely pharmacy assistant said, "Look if you're not happy, you can bring it back."

Smart way to get rid of me. Thermometer in hand, I hit the internet to learn how to do this properly. There are some great sites to help with this, even some of which outline "five simple steps." Who knew! I had to admit I learned a lot. Your BBT spikes when you ovulate and then stays at a higher temperature after you ovulate. So all good, except that to really know when the egg is about to pop, you need to record your BBTs for a few months so you are able to see the pattern and then you can work out when you are likely to ovulate. Makes sense, except that this was a few more months past the thirty-five-year-old timeline, which seemed a few months too many. I didn't want to wear Sam out, so I said, "Let's first figure this out for a couple of months and then focus our efforts on the 'critical time.'" We went back to fun sex for a while.

I can't say I ever really got to grips with my cycle. I had temperature spikes all over the place and none of my charts seemed to match the perfect ones I found online. There would be a more pronounced spike on my Day Thirteen so we decided that that was going to be our target. The other thing, that again I am sure most women know but was a complete surprise to me, was the fact that sperm can live inside you for up to five days.

Think about this. You can have sex … but it's not until you are picking up groceries a couple of days later when wham … you are in the process of making a baby as you stand in the check-out line … all by yourself! Amazing!

It had now been about seven months of trying. We were timing sex around ovulation—measuring temperatures and trying to "do it" every day during the "critical time period." This caused us a lot of stress. Sex now had an end game. Sex was now about creating a baby. Sex was no longer fun. I so admire the guys at this point. Really, regardless of whether they want to or not, they have to perform. Yes, women also have a difficult time, but we can still get pregnant without having an orgasm. Guys have to make it happen. I give Sam full marks on this item. He was a trooper. Not once did he waver in his determination to create a mini-Dexter, even when I knew he wasn't up to it and would rather probably do anything other than have sex with me, again. Not because I was an unattractive prospect; it's just that sex purely for making a baby is different sex. It tends to be quick, tense, and after it you end up thinking, "I wonder if it worked this time."

I was losing heart. We kept trying, but there was no baby. So we decided to take things into our own hands at eight months. Sam volunteered first, saying he would go have his sperm tested to see if there was a problem. Sam's sperm was fine. There were a couple of issues with morphology (the shape of the sperm)— apparently there were a few Frankenstein ones in the batch—but overall, he had so many of them that this was not a problem. In fact, I can't remember how many times he would suddenly shout, "Let's play 'Who's got the most sperm?'" The fact that only one of us produced the stuff was irrelevant to him.

At this point, my part was to shout, "You've got the most sperm!"

Sam: "How many sperm have I got?"

Me: "Over 130,000,000 sperm."

Sam: "Sorry, I didn't hear you."

Me: "Oh, fuck off!"

My turn next. Off to my family doctor who gave me the standard battery of blood tests. There are a few more tests with the ladies, but essentially one of the big ones is a **hysterosalpingo-gram (an HSG is an x-ray of the womb and tubes to see if there is anything "mechanical" stopping a woman from getting pregnant).** The x-ray was uncomfortable, as it involved injecting a dye into the uterus; but compared to having to go into a room and ejaculate into a bottle, I thought it was a breeze.

The other really important test is the follicle-stimulating hormone (FSH) test to indicate how many eggs a woman has left. My reading on the scale they use was six and the doctor said that anything below ten at my age was good. Results all came back "normal." The FSH result was good. My thyroid was about three, which I thought—from my Google knowledge—was a bit high, but the doctor said that in Canada three is considered well within the normal range. After reviewing these tests, the family doctor said that there did not seem to be anything "medical" explaining our inability to get pregnant.

I told Sam and showed him the results. He said, "Well, that's good; maybe it's just timing."

I was not so sure. I wanted to find something we could do something about. We agreed we would give it a few more months then head to a fertility clinic. A few more months came and went, and as I approached my thirty-sixth birthday, we decided it was finally time to admit we needed some help.

I researched several clinics in the area and set up appointments. Sitting in the waiting rooms, you suddenly start to realize that you are part of a subgroup of people. These are people who can't get pregnant—these are the "unfertiles." Yes, I know the more acceptable word is "infertile" but to me being "in" something should be a good thing. Being "in" fertile sounds like it's all guns-a-blazing and this is the most fertile time of your life, when in fact it's the opposite. So I am renaming the whole process to being "un" fertile, as that makes more sense to me. Unhappy, unappreciated, unproductive, unsexy, unfertile—I think you get the idea.

Then came time for the appointment. I know the doctors are the experts, but one thing always amazed me. When they saw my test results, the doctors thought they were telling me good news as they always opened with, "The good news is that everything is normal," but you soon realize that what they should say is, "The results are in. It's bad news. We do not have a clue why you can't conceive, so we're going to suggest a few years of going through an emotional roller-coaster; you'll spend thousands of dollars; you'll experience more heartbreak than you think you can handle; and the stress may take you and Sam to the edge."

What most sane people would do is run for the door, but sane people aren't unfertile people. We say, "Okay, sign me up." It's also a lie when they say, "Everything is normal." You're not normal. Normal people conceive. They are the sane people who would run for the door. Unfertiles are neither normal nor sane. Even if you start off that way, at some point through the process you realize you have lost the plot. I am sure it is just as frustrating or devastating if you get a different diagnosis, but at least you know why, the reason for things being the way they are. The one thing I still don't understand is once you are in the subgroup of the "unexplained" (see correct usage of the prefix "un"—"un" is not a good thing), no one suggests a different route than the one everyone else takes. The unexplained group pretty much goes through the same procedures as everyone else.

I visited several clinics. The books tell you to do that, so I did. You are meant to keep going until you find one that you are comfortable with. This is tough. I was looking for the one that would say, "Here's what's wrong and we're going to fix it. You'll have a baby within a year."

Trouble is they don't. They tell you a lot about the stats of your age, the stats of the clinic, and the cost. Several are optimistic for sure, but I think that is when you have a more definitive diagnosis. A few times I felt like I was taking my car to be repaired. Lots of caveats ... "Well ... we're not really sure what we'll find; could take several tries to find out what is wrong" (read: "Take out another mortgage"), and that same sharp intake of breath before they deliver the final blow: "And age is against you."

For the record, I know my age is against me. If I were twenty-one I probably wouldn't be here. That is not new information. I need new news. News that will help me get pregnant. But again, the unfertiles are different. I mean, if this were anyone else, a car salesman, let's say, would you hand over $10,000 to a man who has told you he may not be able to help, does not offer any warranties, and to add insult to injury tells you you're old? Of course not.

To an unfertile, this is like a red rag in front of a bull. You have your chequebook out before he has finished telling you your chances through some infertility treatments are pretty much the same as your chances of conceiving naturally. You don't care. You want a baby. All your friends have one, so you want one too. Soon, however, you wise up. There wasn't anyone with my diagnosis who got a clear answer and a guaranteed plan of how to get a baby. So I switched tactics. I looked for doctors who were nice, but brutally honest. I eventually ended up at a local clinic with Dr. T. I remember walking into his office the first time. Unlike some of the other clinics that were bright white, very polished, and clinical, Dr. T.'s office was a bit dark and full of files and papers. It felt like stepping into my old tutor's office at university.

He asked us about our "baby-making"—or rather "lack of baby-making"—experience and went through our test results. Sam liked him because he commented on Sam's "amazing" sperm numbers. I liked him because he seemed honest. He actually said that although there were lots of advances in this area, he still saw things that made him wonder if they were advancing at all. Women with virtually no eggs and poor quality eggs produce babies, and women who have excellent eggs do not. Dr. T. also had a good sense of humour, which I appreciated.

"I feel I'm becoming obsessed by this," I commented once.

He laughed, replying, "You've seen nothing yet." He did warn us: "Look, what you're about to embark on is not easy and at times you will feel like you're losing your mind."

I said, "Will you point it out to me when you see that I'm on the slippery slope?" I explained about the stress of the basal thermometer decision.

"A little obsessive," he said, "but not enough to render you insane."

"Good," I said.

Sam was a little more concerned. Mainly because I had decided on the most expensive brand of thermometer, because, as we all know, we get what we pay for. Well, with infertility, let me tell you, this is not the case. If I look at what I should get for all the money spent, by all accounts I should have had at least six kids by now.

Dr. T. went through our treatment options. Depending on age and diagnosis, there seemed to be a number of options. He explained that one of the most common first steps is putting the woman on Clomid. It's a pill that helps with ovulation and according to what I have read, forty to fifty percent of couples who use Clomid conceive within six months.

The odds sounded pretty good, but in my case, Dr. T. suggested otherwise. He said that if I were in my early thirties he would have recommended giving it a go, but, as he explained, every month that goes by is another month lost when you are thirty-six.

Arghhh! Any thoughts I had had about there being plenty of time were quickly being erased as we spoke. So I asked, "Based on the fact then that I am 'normal,' but too old for Clomid, what are my options?"

He replied, "Well, we could try IUI." I already knew IUI referred to intrauterine insemination, i.e. squirting the sperm directly into the womb to increase the chances of fertilization. "But based on your results, and the fact that you've been having sex regularly, I feel the same way about it as I feel about Clomid: each month we try it and it doesn't work—we're down a month. So my best advice to you is to go straight to IVF."

He said one of the reasons was because it was uncertain how I would respond to in vitro fertilization; so the sooner I got going on this, the better. Although one can get lucky on the first IVF, it is often a learning process. It helps in figuring out the drug levels required and calibrating everything going forward.

"Great, so it's a $10,000 test," I said. "Do you offer discounts on the first one?" I asked sarcastically.

"Unfortunately not," he said.

At this point, although it sounded like a complete crapshoot, it also made sense to me. Dr. T. was the first doctor who had been this candid with me. Although I am sure all the clinics make sure the first IVF is as successful as it can be, it seemed to me that until you actually do the procedure, no one really knows how someone will respond to a particular drug or procedure.

The clinic was also attached to a university, so they were doing this for academic learning as well as for the purpose of getting results, and for some reason this made me feel better. Some of the other clinics, and some of the information I had read online, had made me feel it was all about the money.

We were now well and truly entering Stage Two of the Unfertility Journey—what I term, "Medical Intervention."

Sam and I went home and talked about it. I still remember thinking that, although nothing had happened to date, I was going to get pregnant the natural way. But I thought we may as well get all the information we could. Plus, we needed to figure out where we were going to find $10,000.

At this point, my sister called. Since Jane had left Bourne with her Prince Charming, who, in the end, turned out to be more like her "Prince Fuckwit," she had travelled the world, living in New Zealand, Australia, and Prague. Now she was back in London. She had built a great career in event management and had had a blast. She had, though, all but given up on finding her mate for life. That was until one weekend when, at the age of thirty-six, she was visiting Mum in Bourne and, lo and behold, she met Mike. Within two months, they had agreed they would end up together and had decided that Jane would move back to Bourne, as Mike lived there with his two sons from a previous marriage. So by the time she was thirty-seven, Jane was married and a step-Mum. Jane was not so elated. She loved Mike, was trying to make it work with his sons, but wondered how the hell, after deciding she was never, ever going to live in Bourne, she was back in the same pubs she had frequented twenty years earlier. Needless to say, our Mum was ecstatic.

Jane and Mike had been having unprotected sex since they first met, but she had still not conceived. But, Jane had a diagnosis: she had polycystic ovaries. This was a fairly common reason for ovulation not happening, and, hence, getting pregnant was a battle. Not to mention the impact it was having on her mood, skin, and general well-being.

When Jane called me that day, she was thirty-nine years old, and, after having "baby-making sex" for quite a while, she told me that she too had decided to enter Stage Two, "Medical Intervention," in hopes of getting a baby.

She had looked into it too and had been given the same advice as me—go straight to IVF. But listen to this: in the UK, if you meet certain criteria regarding age and health condition, and fall into particular categories relating to where you live—like certain counties (mini-provinces)—the cost of your first IVF is covered. In my sister's case, she was thirty-nine and matched enough of the criteria to qualify for "IVF Free." This was very good news, as, at the time, Jane and Mike were strapped for cash and time was definitely not on her side. I wish they had this option here in British Columbia, as it seems very unfair when you think about it—that the chance of your having a baby comes down to money in many cases. It starts to become an "elitist" option in many ways.

Jane decided they were going to go ahead with IVF. I can't give all the details of her journey, as I only heard snippets along the way, but there was one thing that I still find funny to this day. Due to her polycystic ovary syndrome, over the years her mood swings had always been a challenge for her, and I am sure for Mike. When you start on the IVF procedure, they warn you that, because of all the drugs you are injecting, you can suffer from emotional mood swings. For some reason with Jane, the daily injection of drugs completely mellowed her. Mike couldn't believe his luck. I think he tried to steal some of the drugs so she could continue using them post-IVF!

Jane's IVF went very well. She produced a healthy batch of

fifteen eggs, which the doctors were very impressed with for someone of "her age" and there were a lot of them at a very good grade. So good that they let them grow to blastocyst stage and froze five of them. But here's the difference between men and women. Unlike Sam, who liked to burst into his "great sperm" rant at every opportunity, Jane simply appreciated her good fortune and shut up. In fact with Jane and Mike, although the doctors believed Jane's condition was the main reason for their infertility, there was a slight issue with Mike's sperm. They were a tad lazy. I think this meant that when they were placed in the Petri dish with the eggs, they kind of hung out at the side, not really sure how to approach the egg in the middle. Kind of like an awkward school dance. Unfortunately though, unlike at a school dance, if you don't make your move, you die.

To this day, Mike has never accepted that he has lazy sperm. He firmly believes they were just a little tired on the day of the performance.

Bad news came, however: the IVF didn't work. Even though everything looked perfect, two weeks after the transfer date, Jane got her period. She was sad. She would soon be forty and this might have been her best chance. Mike already had two boys from a previous relationship, but I know it meant a lot to them to have a baby together. They weren't sure if, and when, they would try again.

Misery Loves Company

You know the saying, "Misery loves company." I never in a million years thought this was true. I always believed you should surround yourself with positive people if you were miserable, to allow the positive vibes to rub off. Well, that changes when you become an "unfertile." I'm thinking primarily about my friend Maxine, who had started trying for a baby approximately eighteen months before me. She had already tried many different treatments along her journey by the time I was just starting mine, so it was good to hear from someone else who was struggling. But Maxine's journey took a much more severe turn than mine.

Before I let you know her story, I need to paint a picture of Maxine. She is definitely a character. I first met her at a concert of the rock band Oasis, when they cancelled after only one song. Someone threw a shoe on the stage and they left. Done—Oasis left the building. We had mutual friends, as I recall, and although most of our friends went home disappointed, Maxine and I were outraged that our night was ruined and decided that the only thing to do was go to a pub to vent over several bottles of wine. Maxine is a Kiwi and I am a Brit. You'll find that most people from these two nations think that everything can be solved with a drink. Usually it's several drinks and, by the end, you sometimes even decide that your true path in life is to be part of the next female pop group.

It was the start of a great friendship. When I first met Maxine, I thought she bordered on being a precocious private school chick, obsessed with the fact that she couldn't understand why men in Vancouver didn't approach her all the time; I couldn't either, because she's a six-foot-tall blonde and very attractive by most people's estimation. When she finally left Vancouver, she said it was because she felt too ugly here and it was hurting her self-confidence. So rather than spend hundreds of dollars on therapy, she decided to move countries instead. It worked. She found her husband in the States.

She is also still angry that I never made it to her wedding in New Zealand. This is despite the fact that I had my own sister's wedding to go to at the same time, but she still, to this day, does not see that as a good reason. But that's Maxine and that's why I love her. She is a Princess. The world often revolves around her, but she recognizes her own faults, and has a wicked sense of humour. And she's also solid as a rock when it comes to friendship.

One night I got a call from Maxine. The first thing she said was, "Go pour yourself a big glass of wine; you'll need it." So I did. I could tell she was a bit drunk already and upset. After I had my glass in my hand, she told me, "I found a lump, and it's breast cancer." She was thirty-five. We both just cried and drank. Nothing was said for a while. I asked what stage it was at and she said Stage Two. Stage One would have been better, but Stage Two was better than Stage Three or Four.

The one memory I have of that night, along with the shock and the thought that this shouldn't be happening to Maxine, was her humour. That same week she had also found out that her stepfather had bowel cancer (in terms of survival, a far more serious condition) and she was totally pissed off. Jokingly, she said that the one time in her life when all the focus should be on her, she had to share the family "limelight" with her bloody stepfather!

The more we talked she let me know that it looked like her cancer was quite aggressive, since it was receptive to some or all female hormones. Even though I'm not a cancer expert, I knew that wasn't good. They needed to act quickly and she was scheduled for a lumpectomy the next week. I also remember us both coming to the conclusion that maybe this was the reason for her infertility. Her body couldn't let her get pregnant, as that would not only put her health at risk, but also risk the baby's survival.

She may not have said it, but I think there was some small relief for her in knowing that this was potentially the cause of her infertility, as she—like me—had been in the "unexplained" group. After she got her diagnosis, we were in regular contact even though she lived in the States and I lived in Canada. I think we were a lifeline for each other when the days got really bad. I am not saying infertility is anything like cancer, but having a friend who has experienced part of what you are going through does make it better. We laughed about how she could still have "the upper hand." As the old saying goes, there is always someone worse off than you, and this was true in our case: cancer beats infertility hands down.

We both agreed that the only reason we called each other so often was because we were both miserable and that gave us comfort. We also agreed that we would have to stop calling if one of us got happy, as that just wouldn't work. The "good news" for us was that neither of us got happy over the next two years; so we talked a lot.

When Maxine went for her scan to see if the cancer had travelled, someone was definitely watching over her. This was despite the ridiculously painful process of having five needles with dye injected into her boob. To this day, she winces when she talks about that. Her surgeon, however, did something that day that I think saved her life. Apparently, in ninety-nine percent of cases, if breast cancer travels, it travels to the lymph nodes under the arms. They were clear. For some reason, the surgeon decided to check the lymph nodes in her chest. They were not clear. If he had not done this, they would never have known that the cancer was already travelling.

The results of the scan meant she needed full-on chemotherapy for six months. She called and made me laugh when she told me that Tom, her husband, had said that she had sold him a bill of goods. On paper she looked great: smart, six foot-tall blonde, good sense of humour, etc. Now the truth had come out: she couldn't conceive, and, to top it all off, she now had cancer. He had married a lemon and was looking for a refund. I've always liked Tom. He has to be a saint to live with Maxine.

They wanted to start chemotherapy straight away. This brought up a dilemma. The chemo and post-chemo drugs she would have to be on would put her body in menopause for at least two years, depending on the drug schedule. So what did this mean for her chances of having a baby? Her only real option was to retrieve her eggs before she started chemo, because the body could stay in menopause post-drugs and treatment. In reality this meant that Maxine would have to undergo the first part of an IVF right away so that they could retrieve as many eggs as possible, as in all likelihood these could be the last eggs she would ever produce. The issue was though that the IVF drugs that she would be injecting into herself to increase the number of her eggs would also increase the production of certain hormones, the ones that had likely caused her cancer in the first place.

Her oncologist had advised her not to proceed with the IVF, as in his opinion it was high-risk, bearing in mind her type of cancer. Maxine expected this advice, but she wanted a baby. Time also was not on her side. If she were going to go ahead with the IVF, she had only one shot before the chemo started; she would have to make the decision within the next twenty-four hours. She had a fertility clinic standing by that would carry out the IVF, but there was only a small window for her to get it done.

We chatted and I asked about how she felt about adoption. This was a real option for someone in her situation. She and Tom had discussed this and were at a stalemate. Tom was very firm that he did not want to adopt; he would rather it just be him and Maxine than have to go through the adoption process.

She asked me what I thought she should do. I didn't really know what to say, but I did know that she wanted a baby, very badly. I said the only thing I could, "You know the risks, but I guess this could be your only chance of having a baby. Unless you are okay with living with the potential regret, if in fact you stay in menopause, then I think you should do it."

This was a very hard conversation; we were basically agreeing that she should risk aggravating her already aggressive cancer for the "chance" of a baby in the future. After I put the phone down I hoped and prayed that this was the right decision for her.

Maxine sent me a text the next morning. She had made the appointment at the fertility clinic. Again, I don't know if fate was playing a part, but being in Colorado at the time was very lucky for Maxine. Colorado not only had one of the most respected and successful cancer clinics, but they also had one of the most successful fertility clinics.

When I got the next call from Maxine, she was in tears. They had driven the two-and-a-half hours to the fertility clinic, met with various doctors, and then were told that the timing was just too tight before the chemo. They needed to start the treatment on the Monday, but unfortunately it was a statutory holiday, and they just couldn't make it work. I think Maxine felt her world collapsing at that point. She had agonized over the decision, had got Tom on board (he was rightly much more concerned about her beating the cancer than about having a child), only to be told that it wasn't going to happen. This meant that she most likely had to say goodbye to her dream of a family. She and Tom got in the car and headed back home to pick up the pieces, and to try and figure out how they were going to get through the next while.

About an hour later, I got another call. They were turning the car around and heading back to the clinic. I'm not certain what had fully transpired, but the clinic called and said, "Look, if you can get back here today, we will try and make this happen for you."

They had had an internal discussion and, after meeting Maxine and Tom and learning what they were up against, they had decided that they had to help. To this day, the staff at that clinic probably don't know how much that decision meant; that it possibly saved both a marriage and the sanity of my best friend.

She started the IVF program. The oncologist wasn't happy, but he understood. I think Maxine was just mentally exhausted. In the last month, she had discovered she had cancer, had her hopes of having a family nearly wiped out, and was now starting IVF that she knew could in fact endanger her life. She poured herself a large glass of wine and in true Maxine-style said, "Bring it on." Maxine started on her drugs on the Monday and, about two weeks later, she had sixteen eggs. This was the first good news Maxine and Tom had received in a long time, except that, like my sister's husband Mike, Tom's sperm was also a little slow on the uptake. Tom was a hard partier and, I think, believed that he shouldn't have to chase a woman at any cost. His sperm apparently had the same attitude. They relaxed in the Petri dish, flexed their muscles (or heads) a bit, but refused to make the first move on the egg. Unfortunately, they didn't figure out that the eggs don't actually move, and if they didn't do something, like Mike's sperm, they would die. And that's what happened—they died. So Plan B was needed. Plan B was ICSI (intracytoplasmic sperm injection). Essentially with ICSI, the sperm does not get a choice—the medical team chooses the best sperm from the pack and injects them directly into the egg, whether it wants or not, to increase the chances of fertilization.

So Tom's sperm were spun, graded, and then the lucky sixteen were injected into the eggs. Tom and Maxine then had to wait to see if they fertilized. Thirteen did and thirteen made it to day five, to be called blastocysts. These mini-Toms-and-Maxines were then put in the deep freeze until an unknown future date when—everyone hoped—Maxine would be able to carry her own baby. Little did Maxine know that this was the start of a very long journey; but in her heart of hearts she knew that despite the risks to her health she had made the right decision.

Within two weeks, Maxine had started chemo, was beginning to lose all her blonde hair, and was in the living hell of battling cancer.

The time had also come for Sam and me to make a decision. Despite my somewhat deluded belief that I was not going to need IVF, a time came when it was clear that, due to the lack of desired results, we needed to take the "medical intervention" stage to the next level. So we decided we would be ready to move forward in six months.

Why six months?

I had read a lot of information about how to increase my chances of success with IVF and the choices I could make to help. The first of the big three was to quit alcohol. Sorry, not a hope of that happening I'm afraid—a glass of wine was the one thing helping me get through my unfertile phase. After Googling all the information possible about being unfertile, a nice glass of Pinot Grigio was my best friend, but I was prepared to cut back significantly.

The other two of the big three for me were eat well and try Traditional Chinese Medicine and acupuncture. A lot of people had recommended these therapies, most of them advising that I needed to try them for about six months to ensure optimum results. All my life I have been interested in alternative health therapies, so this suggestion was right up my alley. I know this is ironic when you consider that I was about to embark on a drug-induced, completely non-holistic way of trying to conceive a child. However, I told myself that Chinese medicine was the best of "East meets West."

I phoned Dr. T. and told him that I was thinking of undertaking Traditional Chinese Medicine and acupuncture to try and get my body in the best possible shape prior to the IVF. I was actually curious to see what his response would be as a "Western" medical doctor. He was great. Honest as usual, but open. He said, "I've no problem with that, because I know there've been some successes. Personally, I've not seen any better results with patients who do it versus patients who don't. But if it feels right for you, then go ahead. Just please know that I'll ask you to come off the medicine prior to IVF, because no one knows if the Chinese herbs interfere with the drugs."

"Fair enough," I said. "I'm also going to drink my own urine and sit in a crystal cave for a month? Okay with that?" Luckily, he got my sense of humour.

Choosing an acupuncture clinic is nearly as stressful as choosing a fertility clinic. First, I dutifully read Dr. Randine Lewis's book *The Infertility Cure* and made a lot of notes. I then researched all the clinics in Vancouver and signed up for one. Finding an acupuncture clinic in Vancouver is an easy task—there is an acupuncturist on virtually every street corner next to the Starbucks coffee shop. I ended up finding a clinic that specialized in infertility and seemed to have a good reputation.

My first visit was pretty much as expected. Someone looked at my tongue, felt my pulse, and then declared that my liver was not great, my kidneys were weak, my circulation was not up to much, and my head was too full. Oh, and that I am a Type A, and that most people who struggle with infertility tend to be Type A. I wanted to say, "Well, you try going through infertility with an empty head and see how you do."

But of course I didn't.

I wasn't sure what to think, to be honest, as it all sounded pretty dire. Really, I was looking for an explanation about why I wasn't getting pregnant and this didn't seem to give me any answers, but hey, in for a penny, in for a pound. The bit I was not expecting was all those bodily function questions. What was my blood like during my period? Was it light pink, dark? Did it have clots? Was it watery? Crikey! I really didn't know. I probably should have expected the questions after reading the book and mentally preparing. But like most women, when I have a period, I pop in a tampon and forget about it until I have to pull it out. Never during my time as a reproductive female have I studied what came out. So Step One was to notice this next time.

"How do I do that using a tampon?" I asked. "It's just red, so I can't really answer the questions."

The acupuncturist suggested shifting back to sanitary towels until we had figured it out. I don't know about you, but it had been decades since I used a towel. I find them uncomfortable and, for me, not particularly hygienic. However, needs must, so back to sanitary towels it was.

Based on what the acupuncturist had discovered so far, I asked him what I should expect from the acupuncture treatments. He said that it should help with stress, which impacts my hormones, and with egg production and egg quality prior to my IVF. All good stuff to an unfertile's ears.

Ten minutes later, I was half-naked, had several needles stuck all over my body, and had wind chime music ringing in my ears. I loved acupuncture. It totally relaxed me, made me feel calm, and allowed me to fall asleep.

I wasn't so keen on the herbs though.

After every session, I would leave with seven days' worth of herbs and I would have to go home and separate the thirteen different herbs into the seven days. And, oh my God, did they taste awful! The first time I tried them, I swallowed the drink and then about five minutes later I threw it all up. I have a sensitive stomach at the best of times. Anyway, I persevered. Every week, twice a week before work, I would visit the acupuncture clinic, often at seven in the morning to make sure I got in the right number of treatments. At various points, I would sit down with the doctor to check in about how I was doing. For the record, my blood was pink, clotty, and a very light flow. Not the best diagnosis apparently.

I was still measuring my BBT and had high hopes that the acupuncture would help make my charts look like the ones I had Googled. It didn't seem to be helping on that front, but I did feel calmer, so I was hoping that would have an impact on my chances of conceiving through IVF.

I usually like to finish what I start, except for diets, so although I didn't really feel that visiting the acupuncturist was making a big difference, because we were still not pregnant, I kept going. But it was starting to get very expensive. Each visit was about $70 and then the herbs were about $40. Having a health plan meant I could claim back a certain amount, but we reached our limit pretty quickly. I have to say though, thank you British Columbia for being open enough to see Chinese Medicine as warranting medical coverage in some plans. It helped a lot and for many women on the infertility journey, it can be a life saver.

Over time, I experienced a few shifts in my body. My boobs were hurting less and my period was less painful. I had always had regular periods, so no change there. My "flow," as they referred to it, seemed pretty unchanged to me, but I clung to the hope that all this was going to be worth it, because when the IVF started I would produce millions of eggs that were top grade.

During this time, I was in touch with Maxine a lot. Chemo was brutal. She had to have it every three weeks. This meant that the first week after the treatment she felt terrible, the second week marginally better, the third week starting to feel normal, and then she would have to start all over again. It's bad enough when you feel sick for a few days, but feeling like that for weeks and months at a time must be unbearable.

Maxine was determined though to beat cancer, as there was no way she was going to let it get in the way of her having a baby. Every day or every other day, she would drag herself to the gym even if it was just for ten minutes, as she had heard exercise would help. She changed her diet to help her body heal during chemo and she started yoga.

She also decided to aim for a promotion at work. When she told me this, I thought she was crazy. Taking on more stress and more responsibility at this time did not seem to be the most sensible decision. She was already doing well as Sales Manager for a top brand hotel group, but Maxine is very ambitious and she thought the opportunity to become a Director in her area would not come around too often, so maybe this would be her only chance. Despite the fact that she felt like crap most of the time, she was determined to go for it.

And actually, the more we talked about it, the better the idea sounded. For one thing, I found out that work was actually helping her keep her mind focused on something positive, versus thinking about how ill she felt most of the time. We had a lot of fun talking about her approach to get the job and how she could use her cancer to advantage. How could they not give her the job? we joked. That would be discrimination against people with cancer. We devised her interview strategy. Impress the hell out of them with her smarts and her dedication, and, if it looked like it was all going south, pull out her trump cancer card and declare that if they didn't give her the job there was a secret PR campaign that would expose her company as a heartless employer. It couldn't fail.

The good news was that after three rounds of gruelling interviews, she got the job without having to resort to the "cancer campaign" tactic. Probably the best outcome in retrospect, but we had a lot of fun planning the campaign.

At this point I will introduce my friend Kari, who had already been trying for a baby for about ten years. She had not yet tried any of the Stage Two medical interventions. This was primarily because both her parents had died of cancer, she had already had a few cancer scares of her own, and, like Maxine, she knew that IVF and the hormonal drugs could raise her cancer risk significantly. IVF was not something she or her husband were prepared to choose. I hadn't actually told very many of my friends that Sam and I were struggling to have a baby, but knowing that Kari had been going through this for a while, I needed another person who could understand what I was feeling. It was back to the "misery loves company" theory, of which, during infertility, I am a huge fan! However, in terms of my friendship with Kari, we also shared a bond by creating some humour out of our situation.

We would meet for a glass of wine every now and then, and bitch about how unfair life was. I would fill her in on my alternative-health escapades, my herb-taking routine, and how important the "flow" was for conception, while she would fill me in on her latest test that showed she was perfectly "normal" and that, despite having sex for ten years at the right time, still nothing had happened.

One day I said, "Kari, you do know when you ovulate don't you?" I was now officially an ovulation-timing expert!

"Of course," she said. "What do you think I've been doing for the last ten years? I ovulate two days after my period."

"Kari, that's pretty unusual, you know—usually it's ten to sixteen days after your period. I think you've been having sex at the wrong time for ten years!"

"Holy shit," she said. "Maybe that's why it's not working."

She looked at me then and I knew she was joking. She, like me, had been monitoring her ovulation religiously for the last while, but I liked her sense of humour and the fact that she liked white wine as much as I did.

One day, Kari announced that she and her husband had accepted that they were not going to get pregnant naturally and that they were going to go the adoption route. I think she was forty-two at the time. She had already started looking into the process and knew that it could take several years and cause a lot of heartbreak. So although there was some relief in the decision, she also knew that there were no guarantees with adoption and that it is a lengthy process that could consume all her energy and a lot of her bank account.

Luckily, her husband was building a very successful career, so she hoped that they would be okay on the financial front. The more I learned over the next few months, the more the adoption process seemed stressful and just as big an emotional roller-coaster as the IVF journey. In some ways, it can be harder; with IVF, no one really assesses whether you are a "good" potential parent. You do not have to meet the requirements of the people giving the baby up for adoption. And the really emotional kicker with adoption is that in some cases the birth mother can change her mind at any moment even after the baby has been handed over. This must be incredibly stressful. You undergo all the craziness to get a baby, yet, once you first have the baby in your arms, it must be very difficult to bond when you know there is a chance that the baby may be taken away.

After exploring all the options, it was determined that foreign adoption was really the only route for Kari and her husband, as they were older. So her first port of call was to find an agency that could represent her and help her navigate through the complex world of foreign adoption. And I thought finding a fertility clinic was a challenge.

A few weeks passed and then my sister called. Jane and her husband were going to try for a baby again. But instead of doing the whole IVF process, they were just going to insert some of the frozen eggs (defrosted of course!). This would mean the cost would be significantly less, as she was not using as many of the drugs and it also entailed fewer medical procedures. She had a good batch of eggs, so they were hopeful.

Unbeknownst to me, my sister was also doing acupuncture, because this is meant to be incredibly helpful with PCOS (Polycystic Ovary Syndrome). I was actually very surprised. My sister had never really been interested in alternative approaches and I was even more surprised that she had actually found an acupuncturist in her area. You may remember she lives in Bourne, a pretty rural town in the UK, ninety-nine percent Caucasian, and a fairly "mainstream" English market town. There was only one black girl in town when I was growing up there, I remember. Her name was Amy, but everyone referred to her as the "black" girl; you get the picture.

And what was even more surprising, based on the above, was that Jane's doctor was Chinese. He couldn't understand her and she couldn't understand him. Luckily, he was very knowledgeable and could tell a lot from just looking at her tongue and taking her pulse, so it seemed to be working out well. She was also doing this in preparation for her second IVF and overall she felt she was getting positive results. After years of irregular periods, she was finally on a regular schedule, her blood apparently was now the right consistency, and the duration of her period was the right number of days. Her mood swings had diminished; again another sigh of relief from Mike. I have experienced my sister's pre-menstrual moods and they are not pretty. I think Mike just goes out a lot when her moods get ugly.

I could tell Jane was nervous this time. She was forty and thought this was probably her last chance. Plus, having to pay this time for the treatment was putting her and her husband under a lot of financial strain. There was a lot riding on this one.

Jane called me after they had "defrosted" the five eggs that she had previously frozen. One hadn't made it, but the other four looked okay. This raised one of the big dilemmas in the IVF world. Because of the fact that with IVF a woman's chance of having a multiple pregnancy increases, there is an ongoing debate about how many eggs should be transferred. At the time of my sister's IVF, because she was in her forties and the likelihood was that this was her last chance, the thinking was that more eggs should be transferred. So they transferred three eggs. I understand that these days fewer eggs are being transferred, basing the decision on a number of factors: the increased risk of health complications for mothers and babies that come with multiple births, the potential strain these births can put on the healthcare system, and also the improved chances of conceiving through IVF. The latter I am unsure of, but I am optimistic. With so many people having to undergo IVF treatment, I bloody hope the medical community is getting better results.

My sister never really spoke about her feelings concerning the whole IVF journey. Jane is incredibly practical, but I knew she was increasingly concerned about how "old" she was getting and about whether she was getting a bit "too old." It didn't help that, in the town where she lived, all her friends had lived there most of their lives, had kids in their twenties, and were now becoming "empty-nesters," all while Jane was just starting out.

She said one day, "Julie, if this actually happens, by the time the kid is twenty, I'll be sixty years old and Mike will be sixty-five! We're going to have to work until we're eighty, and I will be the oldest Mum on record for this town."

I started laughing until I realized the same would be true of me at the rate Sam and I were going. It was quite a sobering thought. I suggested that she leave the town and go live in a big city, where

there would certainly be more people in the same situation as her.
"Helpful," she replied, and put the phone down.

Jane's second IVF failed.

Again, everything had looked good, but no baby. The doctor
said that, just like her first IVF, "on paper," there was no reason
for the IVF to have failed. Although, obviously a truthful state-
ment, not helpful. You have no clue what to do to improve your
chances next time. You are prepared to do anything, but there's
no one who can tell you what that "thing" is. I thought back to
what Dr. T. had said about the medical community not really understanding why sometimes it happens and sometimes it doesn't.

I get it, but when you are forty, have done IVF twice, spent
money you don't have, and then no one can give you answers,
you want to leap across the desk and say, "Well, since you don't
have a clue, how about next time you pay for it instead? Because
if I have to have this conversation again after spending another
$10,000 and going through emotional hell, I don't think I can be
responsible for my actions."

You don't say that of course. You say, "Thanks very much."
You hold it together until you get to the car, and then you shut
the door and contemplate sticking a needle in your eye.

The failure of the second IVF was quite devastating for Jane
and Mike. Although they had approached it with the attitude of,
"Let's give it our best shot and, if it happens, great, and if it
doesn't, we tried," when you are down to your last shot and it
fails, being "okay" with that is a lot harder than you expected it
would be. Hope is what keeps us unfertiles going. Each failed at-
tempt takes away a large chunk of this hope and makes it harder
to get up every day. Jane and Mike had to regroup and start putting their lives back together again.

My IVF was now fast approaching. I was still seeing the Chinese
doctor, had been eating like a health freak, and had actually cut
down considerably on my wine intake. Seeing what had happened
to my sister—with two failed IVFs—definitely had an impact on
me. It seemed to be luck, rather than medical science, that made

a difference, and I was not sure how full my "bucket of luck" was at this point. Prior to starting this journey, I assumed that IVFs failed for a reason that was explainable. Now, knowing that this was not the case, I was definitely less confident about the procedure. I did, however, believe that a positive mental attitude must count for something, so I focused on the fact that I was "normal," only thirty-six years old, and had done everything I thought possible to help make this happen for me. With this in mind, we did our pre-IVF tests.

The Point of No Return

"Houston, we are a go." We met with Dr. T. prior to our first IVF and he took us through the process. As he explained, Step One of the treatment really starts after you ovulate. They put you on a "system suppressant" drug—Lupron in my case—which basically means that the clinic is now "controlling your ovulation." Once you have been on this drug for about ten to sixteen days, the first "official" day of your IVF cycle begins. This is usually on the second day of your period, when they take a baseline blood test and a baseline ultrasound. The blood test is meant to check your estrogen levels, specifically your E2 or estradiol. They need to be low enough to indicate that your system is "asleep" from the Lupron and you are now "in the clinic's control." But, yes, an ultrasound with your period is not a pretty sight.

I have to laugh when I think about my prep for IVF. Apart from the "my body is a temple" approach and my Chinese Medicine treatments, I also thought it very important to ensure that I was waxed and pretty down below. I mean with an ultrasound every three days, my nether regions were going to be on display for all to see. When you think about seeing probably fifteen front-bottoms every morning, usually before 9:00 a.m., it can't really be the most "jump out of bed" job in the world.

I know "front-bottom" is a lame word, but I seriously hate the word "vagina." You know it's a bad word when everyone that has one, or has a child with one, tries to think of an alternative word. For me, front-bottom works, but I have heard some classics over the years: the standard ones and then the more bizarre—"happy flappy," "bearded clam," and "penis pothole" are a few of my favourites. I have found a hundred-and-fifty so far!

My blood work came back normal. In fact, my last FSH reading on Day Three was 6.8. The doctor again said that any FSH reading (the follicle-stimulating hormone) under 10 was encouraging. Nothing untoward was found on my ultrasound, so we got the green light for Step Two.

Step Two involves self-injecting the fertility drugs (mine was Puregon) usually between one and four times a day. My schedule was once per day before 6:00 p.m. I should let you know at this point that injecting yourself does not feel that bad. And according to Dr. T., I was one of the lucky ones (versus the skinny unfertiles who hardly have any fat), because having a little more "meat on the bones" actually makes it easier, as you can get a good "roll of fat" to stick the needle into.

Sam was sitting there smiling as the doctor was telling me this, and later he said, "If that had been me who said that to you, you would have punched me in the head."

He was right, but Dr. T. was a man who was going to help me get a baby, so he could say I was drop-dead ugly and as long as he delivered the goods, I didn't care.

I was still working at the ad agency, so making sure I was home to inject before 6:00 p.m. was always a challenge. Ninety percent of the time, I would just be getting in the door at about five minutes to six. I had to run into the bathroom, measure out the amount the clinic had instructed, and then stick the needle in, all in less than five minutes. This usually meant I had no time to think about "placement" or "angle," so, more often than not, I would wake up the next day with a bruise on my belly from the hatchet-job of my self-inflicted Puregon injection.

I was given a small amount to start injecting on Day One. They wanted to start me off at a lower dosage, as they were not sure how I would respond. On Day One, my E2 levels were 59 and my dosage was 225 international units (IU) of Puregon. I had my next blood test on Day Five. I had to be at the clinic at 7:00 a.m. Even though I live in the city, this was a challenge; but for those people living outside the urban centre, it must mean getting up at four or five o'clock. If someone said that if you got up at four or five in the morning you would receive your most favourite item, most people I know would probably still give it a rain check. But not the unfertiles. We are lined up to get blood drawn and a probe stuck up our nether regions before 7:30 a.m. in the morning.

On Day Five of my IVF cycle, I dutifully turned up at the IVF clinic at 7:00 a.m. I was a bit surprised to find so many others there. I know this seems naive, but when you are struggling with infertility you think you are the only one. Most of your friends seem to be popping out babies, no trouble; but no, you are not alone!

When I walked into the clinic I could see there was a whole army of us unfertiles out there! Fifteen in my group alone. In some ways, this was a double-edged sword. On the one hand, I felt a lot better knowing that I was not the only one; but on the other hand, I looked around the group and got a little freaked out. In my head, I thought I was a young IVF participant at thirty-six years old, but I could see that I was actually one of the oldest in the group. Shit!

I knew my chances of success were between fifteen to twenty percent at my age and, looking around at everyone else in the clinic, in all likelihood only a few of us would be lucky. To distract myself from the low odds, I started making up reasons in my head why the others might not get lucky. Too overweight, too skinny, too pretty, too happy, too positive, eyes too close, thick ankles. You name it, by the time I was called in for my test, I had successfully eliminated at least ninety-five percent of the competition. One thing that did stump me though was how to figure out when it was my turn in the queue.

I asked the woman next to me how the system worked, as everyone just seemed to know.

"Ladybirds," said the woman next to me.

"Sorry?" I said, secretly thinking, "Brilliant, I can eliminate this one too," as I made a mental note of "too crazy" to add to my list of reasons for failure.

"You have to pick a ladybird from the box," she said.

"Righto!" I said, and smiled politely, heading toward the box.

Anyway, lo and behold, she was not crazy, but right. In the box were a bunch of wooden ladybirds with numbers on them and the number you got indicated where you were in the queue. Now, I am all for making the infertile journey easier, but I did question the thinking behind ladybirds. I mean, who was the genius who thought, let's use ladybirds, because these women are having a hard enough time with life, so a ladybird, versus a good old-fashioned number, will make them feel better?

Please. We may be infertile, but I think we can handle a number.

Plus someone needs to do their research. Did no one figure out the irony of using ladybirds? Remember the nursery rhyme:

Ladybird, ladybird, fly away home,
Your house is on fire and your kids are all gone,
All except one, and her name is Anne,
And she hid under the frying pan.

Not the most inspiring thought.

I dutifully picked up my ladybird and took a seat.

I think there are two distinct types of women in the unfertile group: those who like to share and those who don't. I was sitting next to a sharer who proceeded to tell me all the details of her IVF attempts to date. Me—I am a non-sharer. I really didn't want to be a part of this group, so for me, sharing my experience was not an option. Plus, hearing that some of these women were on their third or fourth try was just depressing.

My number was called, so in I went for the blood test. All very straightforward. I had "good" veins, so I'd never had an issue with having blood drawn, but I could see for some women this could be a painful process.

The clinic called later that day. My estrogen count was low. Lower than they wanted. My E2 reading was only 346.

"What does that mean exactly?" I asked.

"Well, it means that there may not be as many eggs as we had hoped, and that we are going to have to increase the dosage amount."

They upped my Puregon dosage to 300 for the next two days and scheduled me in for another blood test on Day Seven. That day, my E2 reading was still low, only 488. Up we went again. I was now on 375 IU Puregon.

Raising my dosage seemed to do the trick, because on Day Nine, my next blood test, I was at 1809. This was also the day I had my first ultrasound.

After the blood test, I headed up to the ultrasound department. I have to congratulate the ultrasound team. They had done their research. Here we had butterflies. No dead children from a house fire in sight.

Dr. T. was at the ultrasound. I was glad I had put in the time to have my nether regions trimmed and styled. I sat on the table, not really sure what to expect. There was a rather large probe covered in cold gel that he simply inserted. I have a pretty good pain tolerance, and by no means was this super painful, but it was definitely very, very uncomfortable. They have to manoeuvre the probe around to get a good look at the eggs in the ovaries and that can take some deep probing and twisting.

Nothing much was happening in my ovaries. In my right ovary, I had three eggs measuring above 11 mm, and in my left there were seven, but all below 10 mm. I could tell that Dr. T. was a little disappointed, mainly because he said so. But he said it was still very early days and we had a while to go in order to see how the blood count would be.

Mmmmm.

I left feeling flat. I didn't understand the whole process yet, but the little bubble of excitement I had felt at the start was starting to evaporate. I am not a pessimist, but I have a very strong intuition and my gut was saying that this was not going well. I phoned Sam and let him know about the first round of results.

He said, "Well, isn't ten eggs good?"

I said, "I don't think so. They will likely not be able to harvest all ten; maybe four or six at best. We have to wait for the blood test to come back, so it could be the fact that the dosage is too low."

"Okay," he said. "Well, let's not panic until we get more information."

During the next four years, I lost count of the number of times Sam said those words.

I should probably mention the impact of the drugs during IVF. I had been very fortunate not to have suffered with PMS to any great extent over my reproductive lifetime. But shooting high dosages of fertility drugs into my system changed all that. Most of the time when I was on the drugs, I felt like I had no patience. I was angry one minute, sad the next, and overall I felt as though I was going to lose control of myself at any moment. I would actually start to play out scenarios in my mind about what I would do while in conversations with people, people I normally got on well with. I wanted to punch people, slap them, and scream at them about the slightest irritation. Playing it out in my mind diffused the situation. I couldn't actually do these things, but if I imagined doing them, it helped. Also, I had to stay in control because I needed to keep my job; fertility procedures are expensive. My role at work was essentially to oversee, manage various accounts, and ensure that teams worked well together to get results. Doing this job while strung out on Puregon was one of the hardest things I have ever had to do.

The emotional effort of trying to hold it all together and actually perform meant that, most days at the end of the day, I would get to my car, shut the door, and just cry most of the way home. I would sit in the car for a few minutes when I got home, dry my tears, reapply my mascara, and go in. I didn't need to do this, but I also didn't want Sam to have to deal with an emotional wreck every night. He would have taken it all in stride and he was with me every step of the way, but I felt I needed to be as strong as I could, because this was just the beginning.

There was one day, which I thought had been a good day

emotionally, when I said to Sam, "Hey, you know I think my body is getting used to these drugs and they're not affecting me as much."

Sam said, "Julie, you just cried through *Just for Laughs.*"

Okay, so I was losing my perspective as well as my sanity.

I was on an increased dosage for three more days and, on Day Eleven, I went in for another blood test and ultrasound. I asked Sam to come with me this time. He, too, was bemused by the ladybird numbers. He was also shocked by the number of women at the clinic during our early morning meetings. It did not pass him by that I was also one of the oldest women there.

"Do you think we've left it too late?" he asked.

"Do you?" I said.

What he was really saying was, "Did *you* leave it too late?" as he had wanted to try earlier and I had said I wasn't ready. That hit a sore spot.

"No, I don't think we've left it too late. I wasn't ready before, and yes I'm frustrated that things aren't happening more quickly. But that is what we're dealing with, so friggin' deal with it and don't make me feel bad. I feel bad enough as it is."

I nearly added "wanker," but as we were in public I didn't think it was a particularly good idea, especially as couples are meant to be pulling together and supporting each other through this.

"I wasn't blaming you," Sam said. "I was just wondering out loud, because I was surprised there were so many younger women in here."

He was right, of course. It was the same observation I had had and it scared me, which probably explained my somewhat-over-the-top reaction. That and the fact that my body was swimming in "don't piss me off" hormonal drugs.

Not many people talk about the stress that being in the unfertile group can have on your relationship. I actually think this should be a large part of the preparation for the journey, as I had no idea how the stress could slowly start to undermine what a couple has built up over the years.

You start off with such hope and enthusiasm when you decide to try for a baby. Then when it doesn't happen, the cracks can start to show. Well, for Sam and me, that's what happened. I am sure some couples sail through this journey intact and stronger. For us, that was not the case.

Once we had made the decision to have a baby, we wanted it to happen quickly. When we didn't conceive after trying naturally, we both got frustrated, because we wanted it to happen, and it wasn't happening. But the frustration was a "shared" frustration: we were in this together; there was no one to blame; we were both just hopeful that it would eventually work out. Once you have both had the tests and are both declared "normal," (or, in the case of Sam's sperm count, "exceptional!") you are still a team.

I am not sure when it changes, but it did for us. The thoughts started trickling in. Thoughts such as: "What would my life be like without children?"

"How important is this for my future happiness?"

"Will we still be as happy with each other if this doesn't happen?"

These were my inner thoughts and these were also decisions we had to make both alone and as a couple. It was each person's life at the end of the day and each of us needed to know how we could cope with a life without children, if that was how it was all going to end up.

Though strange, it is sometimes hard to talk about these questions with your partner. The bottom-line is that you don't want to acknowledge the possibility that kids may just not be part of your future and you don't want to ask what that could mean for you both. I knew what it meant for Sam. He really wanted to have a child. I knew that even though he loved me and would still be with me whatever the outcome, it would likely be through a sense of obligation and responsibility. He wouldn't want to be seen as the asshole who dumped me because I couldn't conceive; but I think he would be filled with regret at not having a child in our lives.

That is probably what scared me more than anything. I knew I couldn't handle waking up every day and facing that disappointment. Sam would never openly express it, but the thought would be in his head. I would know it was there, and I couldn't live with that. Sam was also younger than me and could find someone else, and, at the end of the day, I wanted him (and me) to be happy.

We weren't at the breaking point yet, as we collected the ladybird at the clinic; we still were very optimistic that things were going to work out; but there was no denying that the strain of the unfertile world was starting to take its toll. We had no idea how bad it was going to get.

My ladybird number was called and I stripped down for my ultrasound. It was Dr. T. again. At the clinic the doctors rotated for the early morning shift, so you were never guaranteed which doctor was going to be there. They all seemed pretty good, but having your own doctor there helped.

My egg follicles still weren't doing well. They were growing, but very slowly and were still small. I was on Day Eleven and most IVFs last between ten and twelve days before the eggs are at a good enough size to retrieve. My eggs were nowhere near cooked. The three eggs in my right ovary were still getting bigger, but at a snail's pace, while those in my left were still below 10 mm. "Harvesting" size is usually between 18 mm to 22 mm. This is the trick with IVF: the doctor has to time it so he or she retrieves when the woman has as many eggs at the right size as possible. Luckily, the fertility clinic doctors have been doing it long enough to have pretty good judgement.

There were maybe two or three eggs that they thought could reach the right size. Then I heard that dreaded phrase, "It only takes one."

Arghhh! I know it's true, but I'd been producing one egg every month for the last eight months at no cost, so saying this does not make me feel better. I was going through this in the hope of producing multitudes of eggs that would get me pregnant—not one. One I can do alone, drug-free and cost-free.

So I asked, "What's next?" Dr. T. was brutally honest yet again. "If this wasn't your first IVF, I would tell you that we should cancel to save you some money, but as we still don't know how the eggs will fertilize or what grades you can produce, if you are up for it, I would like you to continue so we can maximize the learning as much as possible."

I wasn't happy, but it did make sense, and as hope is eternal for the unfertiles, I had still not ruled out the possibility that this could work. My blood work results for E2 just confirmed the situation, as expected counts were still low: 3187. The clinic didn't want to increase my dosage of Puregon any further as it was pretty much at the maximum; they wanted to add in 75 IU of Repronex. From what I knew it is a "boosting" drug to help kick the eggs into action. My next ultrasound was scheduled for Day Fourteen. This was beginning to feel like the longest IVF ever.

Sam was pretty quiet on the way home. I had been expecting bad news, but Sam was not quite as prepared and he was noticeably down.

I called Maxine. I mean what better thing could I do when I'm feeling down than calling someone worse off than me. Maxine was sympathetic, but also realistic. "It looks like you're going to have to do more than one IVF, I guess."

"Yup," I said.

"Are you feeling sorry for yourself?" she asked.

"A bit. That's why I'm calling you, to make myself feel better."

"Okay," she said, "Take a seat." She then proceeded to tell me what chemo felt like. "I've never felt so sick in my life. My hair is coming out in clumps. My skin is so dry that it's starting to crack. I can't pooh and have managed to rip my anus, so I've to go and have it stitched up. I throw up at work; I straighten my wig that makes my head itch all day; and then I have to pretend everything is okay and that I can handle the pressure of dealing with cancer and a new job. I go home, collapse on my bed, sleep, and do it all again the next morning. Tom is freaked out that I'm going to die and I'm freaked out that I'm going to die."

"And your point is?" I said.

We both laughed. We knew we were both in misery, but it did the trick. I still felt sorry for myself, but perspective is always good.

"Feel better?" she asked.

"Yup, thanks Maxine."

"Good," she said. "1-800 Chemo Line is always open for business."

"That's good," I said. "1-800 Crap Eggs is too."

The drugs were really starting to take their toll and I was finding it harder and harder to be "normal" at work. Also, work was very busy. We were in the middle of a couple of really big sales pitches and the days were long. One day, when I had been in a meeting all day, I looked at my watch: 5:35 p.m. I was out of drugs and I needed to get to the pharmacy and inject the drugs by 6:00 p.m. The pharmacy was on the other side of town so there was no way I was going to make it and inject by 6:00 p.m. I rang Sam to see if he could get the drugs, as he was a bit closer; but he was in a meeting he couldn't get out of.

Shit. Shit. Shit.

I knew we were at a critical phase of the IVF and I couldn't mess this up. I got in the car and drove like a mad woman across town. There was one main pharmacy near the clinic that we used; they were very well-versed in the drugs that the clinic used. I ran to the dispensary. It was 5:55 p.m. and there was a line-up. I actually wanted to cry. I attribute this to the drugs, the stress of the journey, and the disappointing effects of the IVF. I panicked and asked the woman in front of me, "Please, may I go first? I want a baby and that man behind the counter is the only man who can help me right now."

I realized when I'd said it, how odd it must have sounded. She probably thought he was my husband and we had to copulate right there and then, so I explained it to her more clearly. Some people are just good in this world and she said, "No problem, go ahead." I got my drugs and thanked her again.

"Good luck," she responded.

It was 6:02 p.m. so I knew by the time I drove home it would be closer to 6:30 p.m.: too late. I actually never asked Dr. T. what happens if you are late, as to date I had always made it on time, if only by the skin of my teeth, but I assumed it was not good.

I looked around and my only option was the washroom in Safeway. I didn't have any syringes with me so I had to ask the pharmacist for one. I explained the situation. He gave me the syringes and wished me luck. I ran into the washroom, got very paranoid about needles and hygiene, but, with very few options, had to ignore those concerns, measured out the amount, and rammed the needle in. It was 6:06 p.m.

I came out and thanked the pharmacist for his help. "No problem," he said. "By the way, you know there are security cameras in there, right?"

"Great! Well now, you have footage of a thirty-six-year-old shooting up in your washroom. At least you can help me explain when the drug enforcement team comes to take me away."

"I never saw you," he said and then laughed. "Just kidding, it happens all the time. Hope it works out with the IVF." Funny, funny guy.

I think I hit a new low at this point in my IVF journey. Sitting on that toilet, injecting myself, surrounded by used toilet paper, and god-knows-what on the floor, I asked myself is this what I have to do to get a baby? Why, why, why can everyone else have a baby the "normal" way, when I have to go through this?

This brings up an interesting point. So many people have asked me how to cope when everyone else seems to be getting pregnant and you are not. I wish I had the answer, but the truth is that you have to find your own way through this and it is tough. Many of my friends were thirty-five-plus and in long-term relationships. This is probably the worst situation for an unfertile, as suddenly everyone is acutely aware of their biological clock, and if you're even just thinking about having a child, you're told that now is the time to do it.

Lucy was first. I had met Lucy many years earlier in a work situation. I was her boss and loved working with her. She was passionate, smart, and very determined. An Italian chick through and through. But she was unhappy. All her friends were married and having kids, and Lucy was feeling frustrated that she was not in the same position. She was twenty-eight at the time.

"Are you crazy?" I said. "You're only twenty-eight. You need to get some new friends."

I invited her out to my thirty-plus crowd, who were mostly single career women having a great time. Lucy fit right in and to this day she is one of the seven friends who form my core group. She stopped panicking about the marriage bit and relaxed a little. She was clear though that she still wanted a family by thirty-five and kids were a very big part of this, but at least now she had breathing room.

Once she started to relax, she met James. Funny how that happens. Within two years, she was engaged and planning her wedding. She had been upfront with James that family was critical to her and that she wanted to start working on it pretty soon after they were married. She was pregnant by the time she got back from her honeymoon. I think, even for Lucy, this was a little quick. For James, quicker still.

So for Lucy it took exactly one month to get pregnant. Although I was envious, one friend getting pregnant quickly was okay to deal with emotionally. Plus, Lucy had always been very clear that this was what she wanted, so I couldn't help but be happy for her.

Over the next twelve months, two more of the seven girls got pregnant. We were at a social gathering at one of our friends' homes and this is where my "baby radar" intuition suddenly came into full force. I don't know how it happened, but I suddenly knew that one of the girls was pregnant. Anyway, when one of us isn't drinking (we drink a lot), we always ask that person, "So, are you pregnant?" What other reason could you possibly have for not drinking?

This time, my friend Thalia said, "Yes, I am actually."

My stomach contracted. This is where I had to put on my game face and do what is right. Be happy for my friend and congratulate her. However, there was a double whammy coming at this point, because then our other friend Caroline announced that she too was pregnant. I headed for the kitchen to pour myself a glass of wine and found Kari—my friend who was considering adopting—had beaten me to it. We didn't have to say much, as we both knew how the other was feeling. So we took a big swig, a deep breath, pasted on our smiles, and rejoined the celebrations.

The truth is you are happy for your friends. Truly happy. You are just sad for yourself. Just once I wanted to be the one making the announcement. But these were my friends, so I had to find a way to deal with it.

So, in terms of advice, I have developed a few simple suggestions along the way: find other unfertiles. I found that I could genuinely be happy for my friends, but God, was I glad that I knew at least two women who were suffering as I was. If you don't know anyone, I suggest you hang around the fertility clinics and throw yourself at the first person you think you might get along with who looks like they have been through the ringer. You may have to dump them when they get pregnant and join the "fertile group," but make the most of the misery while you can.

My other piece of advice is this: give yourself a break. When you receive yet another invitation to a baby shower, if you really can't handle it, don't. Most people are lucky enough not to have to go through the infertility journey, so they have no idea about the emotional roller-coaster you are on. If these events completely drain you, only attend when you know you can deal with it. Sam was the one to give me this great insight after I came home from one such event and started crying as soon as I came in the door.

He said, "Look, I know they're your friends and that you love them, but just don't put yourself through it if it's going to do this to you every time. That's why I don't go."

I'd never really thought that Sam was feeling the same way I was, but when he said that I knew he was in as much pain as me.

He's just better at protecting himself. My sense of obligation to celebrate my friends' good fortune was really doing a number on my mental health.

Day Fourteen arrived and I prepped myself for the ultrasound. There had been some movement. My E2 level was now 7021. Two of the eggs on the right side had made it over 17 mm; but only one on the left had. The clinic couldn't let this one drag on any longer, so they scheduled a final ultrasound for the next day and the Ovidrel injection for the next evening. For those who don't know, Ovidrel is the "mother lode" drug. This is the hormone that causes your eggs to finish maturing and get themselves ready to be sucked up a syringe.

I went in for my final ultrasound, with my egg retrieval now to be done thirty-six hours after the Ovidrel injection. The last count stood at three eggs over 20 mm on the right and two eggs over 16 mm on the left. The clinic was still hopeful about getting a few good ones, but we all knew that this was a marathon IVF, so even if we did get a few, the fact that they had been "cooking" so long might have affected the quality.

Nonetheless, despite my previous negativity toward "it just takes one," when you're in a desperate state, you start buying into the "it just takes one" theory, as really, what choice did I have at this point? It was back to the "positive thoughts can have a big influence" approach. I decided this was the route I was going to take. Sam was better when I was positive too. If he saw that I was believing this could happen, he felt more optimistic too.

I didn't tell him that actually I was feeling the opposite. My gut was telling me this wasn't going to work out; I was just choosing to try and give it the best chance I could. Being positive and hopeful was the way I was going to approach it.

Egg-retrieval day arrived. Now, I don't want to freak anyone out here, but they told me it was a relatively painless procedure. Well, I'm sorry, but it's not. It wasn't for me at least. Essentially for the retrieval, they put a needle through the side of your vagina, pierce the ovary and aspirate the eggs on one side, and then they repeat the process on the other. They gave me some drugs to relax me, but within a minute I was asking for more. Whether my ovaries were in a difficult position or this was the doctor's first time, I was not sure, but it bloody hurt. As the tears ran down my cheeks, I was praying that this would all be worth it.

They said they had retrieved a total of six eggs to fertilize. I knew they wanted ten to twelve, but six was what we had. Bearing in mind that they thought we would end up with two, I thought this was good, because in my mind I assumed that all six eggs would fertilize. This is the point at which I think counselling is needed. Before you start an IVF, someone should sit you down and point out all the possible highs and lows of the process. I wish someone had done this with me. But no, that is not the case. No one told me there was a chance my eggs wouldn't fertilize, or maybe they did tell me and I just forgot. But when the clinic called twenty-four hours later, I was not prepared.

"It's not great news," they said. "Two of the eggs did not fertilize at all; and two were 'polyspermic.'" (This term means that eggs are fertilized by two sperm, making them null and void.) "So we're afraid you have only two eggs that are actually fertilized and we're unsure what grade they will be. But we will transfer them in three days' time."

I put the phone down. Although I knew there could be fertilization issues having heard about "lazy sperm" with both Jane and Maxine, I really had not considered the fact that there would be any fertilization issues with *my* eggs. And who knew that an egg could be fertilized by two sperm and that could be a problem? I guess when the quality of the egg is so low, this sometimes happens. Or perhaps Sam's sperm were just overenthusiastic and suffered from his lack-of-communication gene, forgetting to tell each other which egg they were aiming for!

I have no idea what happened, but within the space of twenty-four hours I went from being excited about the number of eggs we had to being in despair, because we now only had what sounded like two low-grade eggs.

I called Sam and told him the news. Just for a bit of background on how this works, by Day Two, the embryos have divided into three to four cells. By Day Three, the lab staff grade the quality of the embryos by looking at them under a microscope. I don't think it is a perfect science and I believe most labs have their own way of grading the eggs, but essentially the grading is done in two ways: cell count and fragmentation. The cells are counted. The ideal embryo has eight, seven, or six cells. If there are more cells than this, the embryo might be growing too fast, using up the stored energy, and therefore more likely to burn out before getting the chance to implant. Fewer than this, and the concern is that the embryos won't continue to divide at all. Also, as the cells divide, they leave fragments behind. Too many fragments suggest that the cells may not be dividing properly. So for example, an ideal egg at Day Three would be an 8-cell, Grade 1.

During this, I was still undergoing acupuncture, but was now getting seriously pissed off with it. So far, it had not helped with the number of eggs nor with the quality, it seemed. I had been doing it for over six months, had given it my best shot, and expected better results. The doctor was not particularly helpful. He said that sometimes this happens and it probably means you have to get the treatment for a longer duration. So what? Another year and another $3,000? Sorry, that's a third of an IVF, and at the rate I'm going, I'm likely going to need a few IVFs. So I said unless there are some guarantees or significant changes, I couldn't justify that expense right now.

However, as I was still in the IVF process, the Chinese Medicine doctor advised me that a treatment of acupuncture right after eggs are transferred can optimize the blood flow to the uterus. I hated this. I had no clue whether this last appointment would make any difference whatsoever; but in the case of unfertiles, if you think there is the slightest chance that this may help, you can't walk away. So I made another $70 appointment for just after my transfer.

On the day of the transfer, I was tired, pessimistic, and flatlining a bit. The news of two potentially low-grade eggs had knocked me over and I think I was still processing it. We turned up for the transfer and were glad to see Dr. T. there. Here though, I have a bit of advice for doctors. Please don't tell your patient, when they are lying down and trying to focus on a warm happy womb for their eggs that "unfortunately, the eggs are not a very good grade and the chance for implantation is low."

My best egg was 8-cell, Grade 4, and the second egg was 6-cell, Grade 3. There was a lot of fragmentation, which probably meant that the eggs were of low quality. Please doctors, tell your patients this information as long as you can before the transfer, not just as you are about to insert the eggs into their wombs! Hearing the information just before the procedure made me want to get off the table and leave. I went from having positive womb thoughts to "what's the point?"

The egg transfer, though, was a much smoother procedure than the egg retrieval. All I had to do was focus on keeping still, so they could insert the eggs into the best place in my uterus. The doctor had a place in mind and used the ultrasound to guide the needle in and release the eggs. All was going well. I was relaxed and Sam was holding my hand. And then suddenly I heard the scrape of chair legs and the next thing Sam was on the floor. The nurses forgot about me and ran to Sam's aid. All the while, Dr. T. was trying to place the eggs in the right place.

Sam apparently felt that watching the ultrasound was worthy of passing out cold. I couldn't believe it! It was *me* on the table having the procedure! Sam was just watching the telly, for God's sake. Mind you, in retrospect, I should have expected it. Sam does have a habit of feeling a little queasy at some of the most bizarre moments. For example, when we went to the opticians he nearly passed out when they squirted air into his eyes, and I caught him pale-faced and shaking when he had to have a heart monitor strapped on to test his heartbeat.

It helped in some way, though. I kept giggling all the way home. He kept insisting that he just got too hot in the room and couldn't catch his breath, but we both knew he was just lying to cover his embarrassment. I just kept thinking—how the hell was he going to cope with a birth?

He drove me to the acupuncture clinic where they were waiting to do the post-transfer treatment. As I lay on the table and had all the needles strategically placed around my womb area, I had an overwhelming feeling that this was not the end of my fertility journey, but just the start. I let the tears flow this time and realized that this acupuncture clinic was not going to get me a baby, and I wouldn't be back.

I was right. Two weeks later, I got my period. I phoned the clinic and asked them if I needed to come in for the blood test. They said, yes, I still had to come in even though the procedure looked like it had failed. Plus, we needed a follow-up appointment with Dr. T. to discuss the IVF and the changes we would make for the next one.

Next one? I could not get my head around that. I went out and bought myself a nice bottle of white wine, had two glasses, and went to bed thinking of the old saying, that things always look better in the morning.

They didn't.

Even though halfway through this IVF I knew things were not looking good, the level of disappointment when I knew it really hadn't worked was very hard to handle. Until the day I got my period, despite the fact that I had hardly any eggs, low quality eggs, and only two that had fertilized, I held onto the hope that despite everything I would still get pregnant. And when I didn't, it hurt.

I was also pretty shocked about how it had gone. If any of my "pre-tests" had shown that there might be an issue with egg quality or ovarian reserve, I would have been better prepared. But the "pre-tests" were all good and "normal." It was even more worrying knowing now that this hadn't been the case. And Google didn't help. I spent a lot of time researching what could be done to help egg quality. Although some supplements were suggested, when I stepped back and tried to take an objective approach, poor egg quality was not an easy fix.

Sam was equally disappointed. He didn't really want to talk about it and kept to himself, but I could "feel" his sadness. This is an issue that starts to emerge when you are going through infertility. To date, we had very much been a team, fighting through this together, and what helped was that there was no one to blame. We were both "normal."

But now that it was clear that the problem was with me, some slight shifts took place. Sam would not blame me and he never did, but our conversation started to change to what do "you" think "you" can do about egg quality and quantity. Suddenly, it felt like it was up to me to fix this. I was okay with that, but it made me feel quite alone. The wisps of dark clouds that had begun to enter our relationship over the last year were starting to build. From this point on, I felt there was a third party in the room. This third party was sad, angry, and very frustrated. He came with us to dinner, the bathroom, and the bedroom. He filled the silences and was often the instigator behind most of our arguments. And he was getting bigger all the time.

I tried to ignore this and at the same time rationalize the fact that Sam and I were starting to struggle. I knew this was common and to be expected. Infertility puts your relationship under a lot of stress and it becomes all-consuming. So I filed these worries under the "Can't deal with this right now" folder and shoved it under the bedroom carpet. Out of sight, out of mind.

Talking to the Dead

I hate feeling out of control, so when I did, I decided I needed to take action. I had to have a plan and my plan was to get some quality eggs. I was back to Google. There is a lot of information out there and despite my earlier dismissal of the information on supplements, I decided that I had nothing to lose (except more money, of course). I set off to the drugstore with my list and, rather than choose one or two, I decided that as I was now thirty-seven I needed to throw everything I could at this issue.

One hour later, I was armed with L-arginine, Coenzyme Q10, omega-3 fatty acids, super greens, DHEA, Royal Jelly, and a pre-natal supplement. Total cost was about $250. I had no idea if these would help. Some studies said yes, some said no, but I didn't care. I needed to rebuild a sense of hope and right now these were the items that were going to do that.

We scheduled our follow-up appointment with Dr. T. This is when the IVF is reviewed and when you try and figure out your next steps. I knew what was coming and knew he would not have any miracle cures, but I needed to hear that he had a plan. He did.

He too was surprised at how badly it had gone, based on my pre-testing. Essentially, he said that it looked like my system was already suppressed and being on the system-suppressant Lupron had suppressed it even more. That could have been one of the reasons why I had responded so poorly and why it had taken so long to get the eggs to "maturation." He said, "Next time, we're going to give you the *old lady protocol*, where we basically skip the Lupron and go straight to the egg-producing drugs."

I asked why my pre-test results had been so good and why they even bothered pre-testing if pre-tests were not very predictive of a woman's response. He explained that the pre-tests are used to indicate if anything obvious is wrong and they can also be a solid indicator if there are problems with ovarian reserve, but, as could be seen in my experience, they are not conclusive in any way.

"Based on what you've seen in this IVF, Dr. T., what do you think my chances are of the next cycle working?" I asked.

"For the first IVF you were in the fifteen to twenty percent success range, based on age and results. Presently, you are down to fifteen percent or less," he said.

Bugger. Bugger. Bugger. That's an eighty-five percent chance of failure.

I told him about the supplements I was going to take. Again, he made the regular response. "I can't tell you not to, but there is no conclusive evidence they work, otherwise we would be recommending them."

But I think he understood that I needed to feel I was doing something that might make a difference, so he was supportive.

He also made me laugh when he said to Sam, "So Mr. Dexter, are you planning any spectacular passing-out tricks for the next one? You might want to practise watching an ultrasound so you can be more prepared."

Sam tried his "But it was so hot in there" explanation, but we didn't hear him.

Sam's male ego was a little dented, "Why did he have to bring that up?" he asked on the way home.

"Because it's funny, Sam—no blood, no needles, no screaming. Just a picture on a screen and you black out. Come on, you must see the humour in that." He didn't.

Sam then coined our new term. The next IVF was going to be the "IVF light"; no Lupron; just the straight goods. I liked his term better than "old lady protocol." We didn't discuss the less-than-fifteen-percent chance of success for the IVF.

The failure of the first IVF really shook my confidence. And I think the "less-than-fifteen-percent chance" had shaken Sam's confidence, because a few weeks after meeting with Dr. T. he asked, "Do you think we should look into adoption?"

I wasn't sure what to say. Adoption for us was definitely an option. And he was right to raise the issue as the adoption process itself can take several years. We might as well start to explore this now rather than wait until after we had given up on IVF.

So I did a bit of digging and found a seminar that was an introduction to adoption. There were about eight couples in the meeting, some young, some older, some same-sex, some not. The seminar began with a brief overview about the agency that had organized the talk and initial steps that you would have to take in the adoption process, and then the speaker introduced a couple who had adopted two children from Africa and had brought them along.

The kids were adorable and I said to Sam, "It's funny; Africa would be near the top of my list of countries I would want to adopt from."

I had spent some time in Africa when I was younger and had seen, firsthand, the impact that poverty and hopelessness has on some of the kids there. I felt that if we could give an opportunity to a child in that situation, it would be an incredibly fulfilling thing to do. Knowing that this child would also fill that missing element in our lives would, I hoped, result in a great fit for both parties.

However, as we sat and listened, I started feeling that I was not ready for this. It was good to know we had this option, but something was telling me, "Not now." Also when we read the literature relating to adoption, it became very apparent that this would be a struggle for us. We were not married, and most of the countries that were open for adoption wanted married couples, and even couples who had been married for at least three years. This totally threw me for a loop. Even if we did get married, we would have to wait for at least three years to apply and then it could take longer than two years to actually adopt. That was five more years of trying to have a baby. I just didn't know if I could handle that. Plus, it felt like the only reason we would be getting married would be so we could have a child. And that didn't feel right either. The more I read, it seemed the best option was for me to apply for adoption as a single woman, but how the hell would we pull that one off when we were living together?

We left.

"What did you think?" I asked Sam.

Sam replied, "Do you think we're going to be able to have a baby ourselves?"

This wasn't what I was expecting. He had obviously been stewing on this.

"Hell, I don't know, but I know I'm not ready for the adoption route. I don't know why. Maybe it's because it looks like for us it's going to be very challenging and just as potentially heartbreaking as IVF. I just don't know."

"But you usually have a good intuition on these things," he said.

I said the only thing I could in response. "Yes, I think we will have a baby. I don't know why. I know the odds look bad, but for some reason I know that adoption for us right now is not the answer. But so far I've been wrong, so you need to figure out what you think too. I don't have any answers."

"I want to keep going with IVF," he said.

"Okay. But I'm not sure when I'll be ready to try again."

"We shouldn't leave it too late," he said.

Arghhh—sod off! I wanted to scream.

I was panicking now. Did my gut really think this was going to happen? I didn't know. I really didn't know, but what was the alternative? To give up? I knew Sam needed to see that I had some faith that this was going to work out. It helped keep him going, but I needed something to help keep me going too.

So when you are completely at a loss and just need a bit of hope, what is the most sensible thing to do? See a psychic, of course. I mean if you don't have any answers, maybe you can get some from "the other side." I think this was the start of my slippery road to insanity. I needed to know that I was going to have a baby and no one in the living world could give me that answer, so now maybe I needed to talk to some dead people.

I asked a few friends if they could recommend any good psychics. One friend of mine—Christine—has always visited psychics so there was a good chance she would have a recommendation. I hadn't told her that we were trying for a baby, but I think she knew something was going on. I hadn't been out as much, and when I was she would occasionally ask me if everything was okay. I would always give the stock answer of, "Work is just crazy busy and I'm a little burnt out." Most of the time it worked.

Christine recommended Gabrielle and I knew that when my friend Maxine visited Canada she had gone to see this psychic. Gabrielle had told Maxine that she would have a baby, but that she had to deal with a medical issue first and the baby was going to cost a lot of money. Little did we know at that point how right Gabrielle would be. Maxine had already been diagnosed with cancer, so she was already half right.

I always get pretty anxious when I delve into the unknown. I love it, because it fascinates me, but when you are sitting there wanting to know something specific, what if the answer from the other side is not what you want to hear?

I asked Christine about this, "Oh," she said, "That's easy. You just find another one that gives you the answer you're looking for!"

Great, I'm sure that does a bunch of good to the reputation of the psychic world.

Anyhow, armed with the recommendation of Gabrielle as a good psychic, I tracked her down and booked an appointment. She surprised me. She was young, trendy, and seemed very direct. A no-nonsense psychic. Not like the stereotypical wise old woman with a scarf around her head. I liked Gabrielle immediately. She was also quite funny when I asked her what it was like to be psychic.

"Oh, it can be a pain. When I was younger all these people would try to talk to me in my head and I had no clue who they were. I thought everyone else heard them too, but I realized very quickly not to talk about it too much, because nobody else was hearing voices. Even today, I have to tell the voices sometimes to go away when I just can't handle them. Plus, I was hoping I would be rich and famous, but so far they've told me that's not going to happen and I have to use my gift to help others. So basically I'm going to be poor, but helpful, and in truth I really don't want to hear that!" She laughed.

"So let's get started," she said. "Before we start I like to do a general reading with the tarot, so just select some cards and I'll tell you what the spirits tell me."

The first card I turned over, was the "mother card," Gabrielle said, "the Empress." Yippee! I thought I had hit the jackpot. This must mean I was going to have a baby. No, apparently not. She said it meant that this was a main concern of mine right now. There were a few more cards that also reflected how I was feeling. Anxious, stressed in my relationship, career good, health okay. But overall, it was pretty good.

Then we got on to specifics. "Am I going to have a baby?"

She turned the card over. "Mmmmm. I think so," she said, "but it may take a while."

I asked, "Is it going to be natural?"

She turned another card over. "It's not completely clear, but I think you will need some medical intervention."

Okay, I was done. That was all I needed to get back on the "hope" wagon.

"Do you have any other questions?" she asked.

I had a few and asked them, but, to be honest, I didn't really care about the answers. I still sat there, however, while she told me I had to get my Candida levels checked, that sometimes Sam was like a heavy weight around my neck, and that written and verbal communication was a key part of my career.

I paid her $45 and to me it was worth every penny. Although, I'm sure she perhaps knew what I wanted to hear to keep me going, and that maybe this is what "the dead people" had told her. I didn't care. I had some hope.

I phoned Sam. "Hey," I said, "I know we have low odds, but I think this is going to work out."

"What makes you think that?" he asked. "Oh, just a feeling I woke up with," I lied. Sam would have seriously questioned my reasoning if he knew I had consulted a psychic. Some things are better left unsaid.

We knew we had to start thinking about IVF Number Two at some point. In order to be able to compare notes, I decided to keep a brief summary of the results of IVF Number One, in the hope that the next one would be better. It did not make good reading.

IVF #1

Suppression drug: Lupron 10 days
Fertility drug: Puregon—a ridiculously long 15 days
Eggs: 6
Fertilized: 2
Grades: Terrible: 8-cell, Grade 4; 6-cell, Grade 3
Result: A big fat negative
Cost: $10,000 + $3,000 + wine
Insanity scale: 4 out of 10—only strayed into talking to dead people toward the end.
Relationship: At start of IVF: 8 out of 10; at end of IVF: 5 out of 10.

Insanity Starts to Take Over

It took me eight months to muster up the courage to try again. This was partly because I wanted to give the supplements time to start working, partly because we needed to figure out the financing, and partly because I just needed time to get ready again mentally.

I had read everything I could about improving egg quality and response, and I was now entering what is best described as my "extreme alternative phase." There were no medical cures that really passed muster in my mind regarding guaranteed results for egg quality, so it was time to try something new.

Unfertiles like me need to feel that they are doing something, anything, in fact, to improve their chances. All you need is one story of how it worked out for someone else and you are ready to give it a go. I actually gave many things a go that I hadn't even heard about before, but the pressure was mounting and there was one thing that I knew I couldn't handle. If at the end of all of this we still had no baby, I needed to know that I had given it my all so I could walk away with a clear conscience. I also have a strong predisposition to the holistic world so this was a scary combination.

For some reason, the thought popped into my head that maybe it was my "energy" that was affecting my chances of conceiving, and hindering my ability to produce good quality eggs.

I had had a Reiki session a few years earlier and remembered that it had a very calming effect on me. It had helped with some issues I was having at the time. So this was my new starting place.

After spending some time researching the "perfect" Reiki person, I landed on Sarah. There are some people you meet in this world who just seem to radiate goodness. Sarah is one of these people. She was in her late fifties and had the most amazing blue eyes. It's hard to explain, but she just seemed to glow. But the good news was that she was not flaky. She was genuine and had a good sense of humour.

We talked quite a bit at the start. She wanted to know why I was there. "I want a baby or at least I want to know why I can't have one. I want to figure out if there's some reason for my infertility other than a medical one. I have old eggs apparently and there is not a lot the medical world can do about that. So here I am."

"Okay," she said. "I certainly can't guarantee you a baby, but I'll do my best to check out any energy blocks that may be stopping your body from getting the results you want."

Fair enough, I was beginning to accept that there is nothing in the fertility world that can be guaranteed, except financial and emotional stress!

So we got to work. Reiki is interesting. Often the "master" does not even touch you. They just move their hands over your body very lightly, shifting and reading the energy. Sarah's hands were on fire. I couldn't believe it: they were red hot and she kept shaking them every few minutes. I asked her what she was doing and she said, "Well, I move the 'more negative' energy, and if I don't shake it off myself, I can sometimes take it on!"

Crikey! I guess this is one of the downsides of the job. I was also a bit perturbed at how often she was doing this. Obviously I had quite a bit of negative energy to get rid of. Mind you, I would challenge anyone who made it through the infertility journey without collecting some negative baggage along the way.

She suddenly asked, "What are you seeing right now?"

I must admit I was a bit taken aback, because at that precise moment I saw an image in my mind of a very grubby and very angry little girl. She was wearing a ragged white dress and had her arms crossed. This chick was seriously angry at the world.

Sarah asked me to approach the little girl in my mind. I had a choice at this point. I could say, "Hey this is not for me" and "Thanks very much," and collect my things. Or I could decide to keep going. I had paid for the session, so I thought I might as well see where this was going.

The funny thing was that every time I tried to get near this funny little girl, she just ran away or threw stones at me. It was very strange. This went on for some time and then Sarah said we needed to move on and come back to her. The rest of the session was uneventful compared to that, but my body felt much lighter at the end and I definitely felt more at peace. Could a glass of wine have the same effect? Probably, but I definitely knew that wine would not get me a baby.

I was intrigued by the little girl. "Who is she?" I asked.

"Who do you think?" Sarah said.

I got it. "You mean she's me?"

"Yes," she said. "Or at least a part of you that has been neglected or not dealt with properly. You need to deal with her, as I'm sure it's not helping in your quest for a child. I'm not saying that she's the reason for your infertility, but sometimes your body won't let things happen until you deal with some past, unresolved emotional issue."

I wasn't sure about this. Yes, I had certainly seen the little girl and can describe her still today, but even for me this was feeling like a bit of a stretch. But hey, this could be something that was stopping me from having a child, so I booked another appointment. I didn't tell Sam about this either. Supplements—I knew he would understand; talking to imaginary little girls in my head—not so much.

Over the next few sessions, the little girl kept popping up and eventually she let me approach her. She was also very sad. There was one session where I couldn't stop crying, as she told me that she had always felt on her own and that no one really loved her. I am not going to go into my childhood background too much, but there were some things she said that made sense to me. As a kid, I lived very much in my own head and struggled with some issues of feeling unloved, probably the same way many people feel. Over time, it was interesting how the little girl became happier and her clothes became cleaner, and she would even hold my hand and take me for walks. Now before you close the book and think I am completely out to lunch, it gets even more bizarre.

One day, Sarah said, "I think you're reconnecting with yourself as the little girl, but I think there's something else, too. I'm going to try something different today, so just be prepared and go with it while you can."

I had been "going with it" so far, so I had nothing to lose. She started working on me and again, just when an image appeared in my head, she asked "What are you seeing?"

"I'm in a dungeon and I'm chained to the wall." Told you it gets even crazier.

"Are you alive?" she asked.

I knew instantly that I was dead.

"Go back five minutes," she said.

Don't ask me how, but I managed to do this.

"What's happening?" she asked.

"I'm holding some rosary beads and someone is coming into the dungeon. They stabbed me in the heart."

"Keep going," she said. "Where are you now?"

"I'm in a car under water." Seriously, the images I was seeing in my head were so crystal clear that I could probably draw them today.

Again, "Are you dead or alive?"

"Dead."

"What happened?"

Same deal, I could go back in my mind. I was in an orange mini car. It was the Sixties. I had a striped scarf on; I was in my late twenties, and I knew I had just taken my own life.

"Keep going," she said, "We're not there yet."

This was definitely not a traditional Reiki session but, hey, on a quest for a baby, who cares!

The next image I had was of me in Egypt, in a temple. I was crunched up on the floor, crying, and bleeding heavily from my "front bottom." I was very sad and angry.

"Dead or alive?" she asked.

"Alive, this time."

"Go back again," Sarah said. The next image I had was of me lying on a slab of stone, with chains around my ankles, and a man—who I think was my husband in that life—was aborting a baby from me. I didn't know why. All I knew was that it was excruciating and that I wanted that baby with all my heart.

I was sobbing at the end of the session. "What the hell was that all about?"

"You just went through several past lives. I felt there was something that your body was holding onto. It was scared about getting pregnant, so I wanted to explore why. The last life we got to may have something to do with it. Your body is scared that if you get pregnant the baby will be taken away."

I really didn't know what to think. But the images I had seen were very clear and maybe, just maybe, there was something to it.

"Do you think I will conceive now?"

"Not sure," she said. "But I feel that your body has started the process of letting go of anger and fear." She also said she got a message that the number eight is important in terms of when I would conceive.

I drove home. Did I even believe in past lives? Probably, I do, as I struggle with understanding how "I" or my soul, or whatever I believe it's called, just stops existing when my body dies. But was this really going to help me get a baby? When I returned home, Sam asked where I had been.

"For a massage," I lied. In my extreme alternative phase, I tended to lie quite a lot to Sam. I justified it by convincing myself that he wouldn't care if it resulted in a baby.

I was probably a seven out of ten on the insanity scale at this point. The medical explanations were not working for me, so when one rational door closes, you do what most unfertiles do, keep opening other doors until you find the jackpot.

What stuck in my mind though was the fact that Sarah had said "conceive" and "the number eight."

For me, this was hope that it was going to happen. That night I suggested to Sam that we try the IVF in August.

"Okay, why August?"

"Just because I think it will be a good month."

"Fine, let's book an appointment to see Dr. T."

Yay! August is the eighth month. This time it was going to happen! We booked a weekend in Naramata in the Okanagan Valley for right after the results would arrive. This would either be to celebrate or commiserate. I just knew I would need to get away.

I had four months to prepare. I would be a mother at thirty-eight if this worked out.

Out of my seven friends, three were now pregnant or mothers, one had cancer, and one was looking to adopt. Debbie was number four.

Debbie was in a completely different situation. I recognized as soon as I first met this awesome gal that she has been driven by the need to create a family. It was, and always has been, incredibly important to her. If she could have her way, she would have lots of kids, lots of parties, and lots of wine! But things had not quite turned out as expected. I think until about ten years ago she saw her life turning out similarly to how the rest of us saw ours. Meet someone, fall in love, and have kids. Well, for Debbie that someone was a woman.

When Debbie finally "came out," we were all super supportive (well, at least, I hope we were). But I often think that must have been really scary for her, as you really don't know how your friends will react, especially because Debbie had some great guy friends and I think she was a bit apprehensive about how it would affect her friendships with them as well.

No surprise; everyone took it in stride and really nothing changed. But this obviously had an impact on the issue of having a baby. Debbie entered a relationship with Angela, a woman who was older and really didn't want children. Angela felt she was past the age of having or wanting kids in her life. Debbie had other plans, and when she decides something, she goes for it. Often I think she would plunge into decisions before thinking everything through, but perhaps in some ways this is better than procrastinating.

The decision was made. Debbie was going to have a baby. The question was how was this going to happen? She needed some sperm. Debbie had two gay guy friends, Chris and Ray. Chris was also keen on having a child. Unfortunately, Ray, like Angela, was not onboard.

Debbie and Chris devised a plan. Chris would "donate" his sperm and he would be involved in the child's life, but Debbie would have full legal rights. This was important because Debbie was from New Zealand and if she ever decided that she wanted to go back home, she needed to have full legal parental rights. If Chris were a full legal "guardian," this would not be possible; Debbie and the child would not be able to move back to New Zealand.

I have to give it to Debbie: she went about this in a very business-like way and had a legal document written up, which both she and Chris signed, before beginning the process. Needless to say, Ray and Angela were not that supportive. Understandable really, as they must have felt that their opinions didn't count. But often the need to have a child means that everything else takes second place.

Debbie, like me, didn't really know how ovulation worked. I hadn't filled her in on all the problems Sam and I were dealing with, so I didn't want to appear to be the "expert." We went for a drink and she said, "I had no idea about all this." Like me, she knew the basics, but having to track temperatures and cervical mucus was a new deal. The good news was that it looked like she was pretty regular and her temperature chart looked okay.

"How is it going to work?" I asked. "Are you planning to have sex with Chris?"

"Julie, he's gay. I really can't imagine that the thought of having sex with me is going to do it for him, do you?"

Fair point.

"The plan is that when it is 'the time,' he does his thing, runs it over to me, and I insert it." Chris lived in the same apartment block as Debbie, so this was very handy, because I don't think sperm are that good at travelling, unless of course they are travelling in a nice, warm "happy flappy."

"When are you planning on trying?" I asked.

"I'm doing acupuncture right now and taking all these disgusting herbs, so I need to give it a few months to let this stuff work."

"Who are you going to?" I asked casually, making a mental note that if acupuncture treatments worked for her I would add her acupuncturist to my list, because I was not going back to the first one. She let me know the name of the person and I scribbled it down when she went to the washroom.

Four months later, Debbie was ready to try. After the event, I asked her how it had gone. "Interesting," she said.

"How did you insert the sperm?" I was curious.

"Turkey baster," she replied.

"No way!"

"Yup," she said.

It didn't work that time or the next. It then became too stressful, I think, for Chris and his partner Ray, so Debbie had to come up with Plan B. She needed another way to get a baby.

Sperm banks proved to be the answer. Debbie did her research and although this was not her ideal method, it really was her only option. She was thirty-eight. We had a girls' weekend away and Debbie brought over details of the potential sperm donor "candidates."

I must admit that it was fun reviewing them. Debs had a shortlist, and the rest of us had to review and give our opinions. I was amazed at the detail provided. They gave us everything from age and SAT scores, to family background and genetic information. They were mostly students. Students need money, and sperm donation is an easy way in Canada of making a few extra dollars. They were a smart and good-looking bunch.

"Don't you wish you could actually sleep with them?" asked

one of our single friends wistfully, after a glass or two of wine. Debs gave her one of her "stupid question" looks.

My vote was for the artistic one. He was very cute, smart, and, from his picture, had lovely forearms, which is a weak spot of mine. Jo's favourite was the engineer. She likes blonds. We knew it was serious stuff, but how many times in your life are you going to sit down and review potential "father" candidates for your gay friend's child? We all fought for our guy and debated why he should be the one, but I think Debs had already made her choice. She never told us which one he was, but I don't think the artist made the cut!

The clinic that Debs was working with seemed really great—helpful and professional. They ordered the sperm and put it on ice for when she was ready.

Sam and I went off for our visit with Dr. T.

"Ready to go again?"

"Yup," we said.

"Let's do the standard tests again, just in case we missed anything."

"IVF light" was off to the races.

Now is probably a good time to talk about money. Each IVF for us was roughly about $10,000—$5,000 for the procedure and $5,000 for the drugs. We were incredibly lucky, because Sam's company healthcare scheme allowed us to claim back on the drugs, up to a limit. We knew this IVF would take us to the limit, so we had our fingers doubly-crossed. The rest of the money we either put on the credit card or on the line of credit. We were both earning at the time so we knew we could pay it off, eventually, but it was still stressful adding more debt to our already growing debt.

That said, we also knew we had very little time left, taking into account my "reproductive" years, so going into debt was our only option. Waiting to save up the odd $10,000 would mean delaying the IVF even further, and based on the results of the first one, when my egg quality was "less than desirable," I didn't think I should risk waiting.

My blood work came back frustratingly normal. In fact, my FSH count was even lower at 6.3, which, if it actually meant anything, should indicate that my ovarian reserve was in pretty good shape. After IVF Number One, I now knew that this meant nothing.

My thyroid count again caught my eye; it was 4.8. I raised this with Dr. T. and again I got the same reply as I'd had from my family doctor when I had asked her about it during one of my regular checkups. This number was within the normal range for Canada: 0.38 to 5.5; but it still felt a bit high for me. I knew 4.8 was within the range, but I was still battling with the knowledge that, according to the rest of the Western world and my mate Google, this is considered too high. Everywhere I looked (and let's face it, I pretty much had been scouring the Earth for the "answer"), it seemed to indicate that anything above 2.5 could be an issue when trying to conceive. It's hard to challenge the medical system though when they firmly believe that the data and research they have is gospel, and you are just one person saying you have a hunch that this could be a problem. I think if I had collected and presented all the medical research from Europe and the States, they might have listened. However, when I was trying to hold down my job, to get ready mentally for the next roller-coaster ride, and to ignore the fact that my relationship was starting to get into big trouble, there was very little time left in the day to do a thesis on why the Canadian thyroid scale might need reworking.

So we took Dr. T.'s input and kept going. One thing though, my Google searches had led me to another potential "cure": meditation.

I kept reading that stress is an inhibitor to conceiving. A woman's body has to be "welcoming" and "ready" for conception. I had quite a bit of stress in my life, so I thought that maybe this was a key factor in my inability to conceive. At first, I tried sitting still and clearing my mind. I put on relaxing music, comfy pants, made sure Sam was not around, and sat still. This was hard. First,

I realized my mind probably had never sat still and I likely went into a state of shock, because suddenly I had so many thoughts in my mind. It was like it was on panic mode, "She's going to shut me down, so I better throw everything I can at her."

My head was starting to hurt and all the thoughts were stressing me out. They switched from my infertility journey, to things I needed to do at work, to all the things that needed doing in the house. Not for one second was my mind still. In fact, for me it was less stressful to actually get up and start doing some of the things I had been thinking about. My first meditation session lasted about three minutes before I gave up. But I am not a quitter, so every day I got up before 6:00 a.m. to give it another go. By the end of the week, I was exhausted and fed up with my lack of progress. Sam would wander in, see me outstretched on the carpet (likely with a frown on my face due to the concentration), casually ask how it was going, and leave the house before I had a chance to answer.

I was starting to get resentful too. It felt like it was all on my shoulders to try and create this baby. Sam never said so, but I could feel his frustration growing and it was starting to seep through in his communication. It was subtle, but it was there. There were more questions like, "Why do you think your eggs are old?"; "Maybe you should cut down on the wine?"; "I found out this supplement might help. Why don't you try it?"

Maybe he was genuinely trying to be helpful in the process, but every time he made one of these comments, it was like a paper cut: it stung just enough to draw blood. My reaction didn't help either. When I think I am under attack, I fight back. It usually came out something like this, "Sam you can always leave me and find someone with younger eggs, you know. Don't feel the need to stay just out of guilt." Sometimes I would add for the hell of it, "And don't worry, I will find someone else. Despite my advancing years, I'm sure some loser out there will feel sorry for me."

I know it was childish, but when I am feeling vulnerable, I have to protect myself. And sometimes I just wanted to hurt him. I was the one that had to have needles stuck in me, up me, and through me; I had been strung out on medication; I had spent hours of my life researching possible explanations for why I was still barren; all to be told that my eggs were old and it was my fault we weren't getting pregnant. Asking dumb questions and suggesting I cut down on wine was asking for trouble.

My self-directed meditation was also not working out. After two weeks of very early mornings and very little sleep, I needed help. I went to the local "hippy, alternative" shop, just down the street. I needed someone to guide me through meditation so at least I could focus on listening to another voice versus my own meandering thoughts. Low and behold, there are lots of fertility-meditation CDs out there. In fact, there was too much choice.

They all focused on very positive, spiritual language: "the fertile soul," "visualizing pregnancy," and "becoming fertile."

I ended up buying a "calm the mind" CD and one that focused specifically on fertility. I liked the "calm the mind" one. There were some helpful visuals created for me, such as slowly descending the stairs and putting all my worries in a box to clear my mind. The only thing I struggled with was trying to get all my worries in the box before the moderator moved on. He obviously didn't have too many concerns going on in his world. I managed to get through this by putting this part of the meditation on fast forward. It was probably the opposite of what I should have been doing, as now I had to ignore the slow walk down the stairs, and instead I ran and skipped to deposit my worries in the wooden box. A little bit stressful, but I realized I couldn't relax for the rest of the meditation if I had not completed this part. I played this meditation every night and often would fall asleep while listening to it. In my mind this was a winner, because over the course of this journey, I was increasingly having sleepless nights.

I did not connect with the other fertility meditation as much. I found the woman's voice irritating. I don't know what it is in the world of infertility, but there seems to be an unwritten rule that you have to deal with the unfertiles with a cloyingly empathetic voice. I also found the language of this one quite depressing. It talked about having barren and cold wombs. I tried it several times, but found myself getting either annoyed or depressed. I know a lot of women had had success with this particular CD, which was why I was so disappointed, but I could tell this was not going to work for me. So back to the bookstore, where I eventually found a CD that focused on the individual steps of the IVF process. Having been through IVF once and now knowing the emotional stress points of the journey, I felt that this would be of better use.

Visualization Part One: Producing lots of healthy eggs. Every night I would focus on my beautiful ovaries bursting at the seams with lots of healthy eggs. We would focus on blood flow, pinkness, and general positive thoughts. Bags and bags of eggs were the goal. I was actually pretty good at the visualization; it came easily to me. I could conjure up, in a flash, images of a pair of heavily laden ovaries with a lovely pink glow all around them.

Occasionally Sam would ask how it was going. "Fine" was usually my answer. I don't think he knew what an ovary looked like, so in truth he couldn't be a great help in the process. The woman's voice was again a bit annoying, but I managed to work through this. I did this every night for two months before the start of my second IVF. By the time I went in for my blood test, I had visualized my ovaries to such an extreme that I felt like I was dragging two potato sacks of eggs around with me everywhere I went.

The good news was that the ladybirds were still there at the clinic. The group at the clinic this time was a lot smaller than the first time. The other patients were still mainly younger than me, but, unlike the first group, there were definitely a couple of "old ladies" like me. One couple really intrigued me. They were a lesbian couple; one was producing the eggs and the other was going to carry the baby, so they each had a part in the baby-making process.

It is quite remarkable when you think about how far we, as a society, have come in terms of the "accepted" ways to have a child. I asked Dr. T. about this one day, about how it all works when it comes to who owns the eggs if any are frozen.

"To be honest, the legal side of these kinds of situations is an unprecedented area," and one which, he guessed, was going to change rapidly moving forward.

"I can only focus on helping people get babies and I'm going to have to leave the legal issues to the legal profession to sort out," he said.

Fair enough. I needed him to focus on helping me have a baby.

My blood work was good, so it was time to start injecting. Since I was doing "IVF light," I skipped the Lupron; I hoped my ovaries would respond better. Last time, they had started me on a lower dose of Puregon; this time they decided I would start on a higher dose, at 275 IU.

It is hard to explain how I felt going into IVF Number Two. Number One had been very disappointing; I just wasn't expecting the poor result. Neither were the doctors! The confidence I had felt beforehand, thinking that this was all going to work out, had definitely taken a hit. Knowing that egg quality was the issue, and that perhaps there was nothing the doctors could do about that, increased the pressure. I asked Dr. T. whether he had a sense of how many times it would potentially take for IVF to work based on the results of IVF Number One. He said that ultimately it was my choice in deciding how long I wanted to keep going, but statistics showed that the chances of conceiving after three or four tries were low.

"Yes," he said, "You will hear lots of stories where on the eighth try it worked, but those are in the minority. You are already down to less than a fifteen-percent chance of success and so, to preserve your sanity, I advise that you seriously consider other options if we do three or four with no success."

Ha! He had no clue that I had already lost my sanity. I wanted to explain to him that the reason I wasn't getting pregnant was because in one of my earlier lives in Egypt, my husband in that life had aborted my baby from me, and that my body was holding onto the fear of getting pregnant. Yup … no. I needed him to get me pregnant, not admitted.

My fears were starting to rub off on Sam. The unpleasant third party that accompanied us everywhere was making his presence known even more. Infertility, which had started off as a small part of our lives two years earlier, now dominated every moment we had together. Even if we weren't talking about it, it was always there. The most innocent remark from either of us could trigger a row. We were sad and frustrated. At a time when you as a couple hoped that you would pull together, I could see we were not. We would go for nice dinners every now and again, and try to pretend it was all okay. We would talk about everything else, except our infertility troubles, but it really felt like we were just putting our lives on hold. We went on pretending that we would be fine whatever the outcome, that we still loved and wanted to be with each other, but at this point I knew the cracks were getting a bit too wide and there would come a point when we couldn't step over them.

But we kept going, because we felt we didn't have any other choice.

I went for my first blood test at the clinic and waited for the results that afternoon. The clinic called. It looked like the new protocol was working—my E2 reading was a high 2265! Woohoo! In fact it was so high, they dropped my Puregon dosage down to 200 for that day. They also wanted me in for an ultrasound the next day. I was hopeful that the high E2 number indicated that there were lots of eggs this time. I phoned Sam. He was relieved, and despite the fact that you try so hard not to get too excited, I couldn't help but start to feel that maybe, just maybe, our luck was turning.

Going into the clinic the next day, my E2 levels were still rising, now at 3042. I was cautiously optimistic. So was Dr. T. He had seen the blood results and was eager to take a look at the ovaries.

At this point, I was thinking that all the "meditation" techniques were paying off, my visualization of heavily laden ovaries might be working!

The bad news for Dr. T. though was that after so many people were checking out, looking up, and probing around my "front bottom," care of my nether regions was slipping. Maintenance was never my strong point and I had in fact lost interest in keeping things neat and tidy down there. It was too much of an effort and to date, no baby. So what was the point?

I got up on the table, slid my bum down to the edge, gritted my teeth as the gel was applied on the probe, and patiently waited for news. It took a while for Dr. T. to say anything. I knew then that this probably wasn't good news. My stomach clenched as I prepared myself for what he had to say.

"There may be a few more eggs, but the bad news is that you have a large lead follicle." This meant that one egg was much bigger than all the rest and that was why the estrogen results had been higher. It was not the fact that there were lots of eggs; it was just that I had a monster one and a few smaller ones. My right ovary had the monster one—it was already at 21 mm. There were three others at about 12 mm and about three at less than 9 mm. The left ovary was again a little slower, like last time, with four eggs between 10 mm and 14 mm and two eggs at less than 9 mm. As you have gathered by now, this, although it may sound like a good thing, is in fact problematic. With a lead follicle, the other eggs are usually quite far behind, so it means that the bigger eggs would likely have to be sacrificed to try and get as many mature eggs as possible.

No. No. No. This was not what I wanted to hear.

"Why does that happen?" I asked.

"We're not sure. Sometimes just one or two eggs 'suck up' all the meds and grow quickly, suppressing the growth of all the others and you just never know if the others will catch up in time."

I was angry. Why was this happening? I always believed that

if you worked at something, eventually it would happen. I had been going above and beyond, and still it was not looking good. Plus it was the eighth month—surely Sarah, the energy woman, couldn't be wrong?

I could see that Sam had called a few times. I ignored him for as long as possible, but I knew I had to tell him.

"It's not good news," I said. "There are a couple more eggs, but the high estrogen levels are because we have a lead follicle." I proceeded to explain what this meant and he just remained quiet.

"Should we cancel?" he said.

"I don't know. Dr. T. wants to see if the other eggs start responding in the next few days, so we'll see." So much for my bloody visualization. That night I didn't do my meditation. You can only keep going so long.

They increased my dosage back up to 250 Puregon for the next couple of days. My E2 was now at 7123 on Day Eight of the cycle. Sam came for the next ultrasound. I don't know why I suggested this. In fact, it just made me feel worse, especially when things weren't going well. I think for us it would have been better if we had lived apart and I had just done the IVFs by myself, not told him any details, and then let him know the results at the end. This way, I could have avoided feeling guilty the whole time and he would have been none the wiser, because it was my old eggs that were the problem. I know that was pretty unrealistic, but I was really starting to feel that this was my journey full of unsuccessful tries. Having to relay the details made it twice as bad.

The lead follicle was still "leading," but the others on the right side had caught up a bit, though slowly. I now had two over 15 mm, three between 10 mm and 14 mm, and the runt of the pack was still struggling to make it to 9 mm. There was one on the left side that had now made it to over 15 mm. Dr. T. decided we should give it one more day, so he scheduled my final ultrasound before the Ovidrel injection the next day. My final E2 count was 10,566 and my eggs had made a Herculean effort. We ended up with four follicles over 15 mm on the right, but only one on the left. The lead follicle was pretty much a write-off at this point, as I think the final measurement was 28 mm. Dr. T. had made the right call in the end. We had sacrificed the big one, but had managed to get quite a few over 15 mm. My left ovary obviously had issues. It had given up at the final hurdle, with only one egg making it over 15 mm. So with a less-than-stellar egg performance again, we were set up for the retrieval. The only good news was that instead of fifteen days on the drugs, this was done in nine! IVF light had its benefits.

My sister Jane called that weekend. She was now forty-one-years old and she told me that she and Mike were going to give it one last try. My Mum had helped out on the cost; she was getting very desperate to have some grandchildren, plus this was one way she could help out. Jane said if this IVF didn't work, they were done. She and Mike had discussed it at length and were in agreement. Mike and Jane seemed to be one of those couples who pulled together; but I also think that because Mike already had two children, and although he was very committed to the IVF, it was different for him. This took the pressure off Jane, too, as they knew they could easily move on together. Jane wanted a child, but she knew that life with Mike could be just as fulfilling without one.

I wanted this to work out for them. Jane had been doing acupuncture all along and felt she was getting noticeable results and that it was helping.

I didn't tell her at the time that we were in the middle of our second IVF and it wasn't going well … again. I am not sure why I didn't say anything. Partly, I just didn't want to talk about it, and partly, I didn't feel that she needed to hear our bad news when going into her final IVF.

"Keep me posted," I said, "and good luck."

"Think about it, Ju. If this works, I'll be forty-two and having my first child."

"Oh well," I said. "The good news is that you have had a pretty interesting life to date, so you can't complain if suddenly it changes dramatically!"

Jane was still on the suppressants, because she is a good responder. When she started injecting, she called and let me know that it was looking good again, just like the other two attempts. She seemed to have a lot of eggs all growing nicely at this point. I was really glad for her and tried to focus on that versus my own dismal egg growth. And yes, I was a bit jealous, but I knew what Jane had gone through and that this was the final chance for her, so I had everything crossed for her.

One time on the phone, I told her about Sam fainting during the egg transfer.

"That's nothing," she said. The doctor that she had seen had made her practise injecting an orange in his office just for demonstration. Apparently, Mike, when faced with a needle and an orange, had the "Sam" affliction and passed out cold. Good heavens! What was it with the male partners of the Selbys? I told Sam because I thought it would make him feel better, but he was just mad that I had told her about his "lapse in manliness."

Seventeen eggs. Jane had seventeen eggs! That was spectacular for an old person! But she had been in the same position before, so she had no expectations. They were taking no chances with Mike's lazy-ass sperm this time, so they fertilized all the eggs with the ICSI technique, when they choose the best sperm and inject it directly into the egg. I always feel a bit sorry for the sperm. What if they picked the uncompetitive one? The one that really wasn't that bothered and was quite happy to be at the back of the pack; who swam at his own pace, and had accepted his fate that in five days' time he would be dead, so he was going to enjoy the journey. Low and behold, he is yanked out of the pack, squeezed into a tube, and forced to impregnate an egg that, naturally, he couldn't be bothered with. And he loses his head in the meantime. I can see why some people think there are more abnormalities with ICSI.

After three days, my sister had eight fertilized eggs that were of really good quality. They transferred three. And so began the two-week wait. Again, it was a textbook IVF (but so was the first one) and that hadn't worked, so Jane was focusing on keeping herself busy until she knew for sure. About halfway through, I checked in.

"How are you doing?" I asked

"Well, I feel fine. My boobs are super sore, but they're always like this before my period—and were like this the last two times—so at this point, I'm not expecting that it's worked." She sounded down, but also said she was glad that after this she and Mike could move on.

I knew she would have her blood test a week later, so I was bracing myself for the call. I was sitting in my car with Sam when I received a text from her. It simply said, "You are going to be an auntie."

I couldn't believe it and screamed so loudly, that poor Sam nearly hit the car in front. I called her straight away. She was the first person, in truth, who had told me that they were pregnant, and for whom I had jumped for joy in response. I would have done the same for Maxine and Kari too, though. Good news means even more when you know someone has been through so much to try and make it happen. I was crying as she picked up the phone. She was too. Apparently sore boobs also means a baby. She was happy. Realistically it was still early days in the pregnancy process, but finally it had worked out. My forty-one-year-old sister was going to have a baby! Needless to say "grandmother-in-waiting" was ecstatic.

I still didn't tell her that I was in the middle of my second IVF. Sometimes you just need to enjoy the moment.

Sam's insightful comment was, "Well, if you have the same genes as your sister, you still have time."

I think this was Sam giving himself some hope. We both knew my IVFs were very different from Jane's. I obviously did not have the "plentiful egg" gene; mine was the "deficient egg quality" gene. But hey, you don't need to mention what you both know. Hope is more important than reality sometimes.

The egg-retrieval day came round and, like the first time, it was extremely painful. My right ovary was a little hard to reach apparently, which equated to twisting the needle a few more times. Luckily, drugs were on hand.

They got seven eggs this time. So I guess the *old lady protocol* was not really achieving greater results than the *young-lady* one. I was better prepared though this time for the fertilization news. Like Jane and Mike, we had elected to go with ICSI, based on the poor fertilization rate last time. It really was the only choice for us.

I told the clinic to call Sam this time with the results. My thick skin was becoming noticeably thin when it came to hearing and delivering bad news.

Four fertilized this time; three were just too old, too big, or too small to make it. "That's one-hundred percent better than last time," Sam said. I actually had to admire his ability to try and take the positive out of the negative. It was a better reaction, so I had to focus on that.

Back I went to my meditation CD, moving on to Part Two, all about creating a welcoming womb for my eggs. I was a little stressed as I realized I only had forty-eight hours to do this, as the transfer was on Day Three. So I doubled up, as I didn't want to leave anything to fate. For the next two nights, I listened to that CD as many times as possible. I had a lovely image of a womb with a cushion of healthy, vibrant blood vessels all working hard to create the perfect environment for my little eggs to embed themselves in.

On the day of the transfer, I braced myself for bad egg-quality news. Slightly better, but only slightly. They recommended transferring three of the fertilized eggs. So my eggs—all 8-cell, Grade 3—were inserted. I remember concentrating so hard on the "visual" of my perfect womb that the nurse had to give me a nudge, as I obviously hadn't heard the doctor say we were done.

Sam as usual was trying to be positive. "The grades were a bit better," he commented on the way home.

"A bit better! The amount of bloody work I have been putting into this, we should have stellar grades. Beautiful little 8-cell, Grade 1 eggs, not fragmented cloudy eggs."

The good news though, Sam didn't faint.

Over the next two weeks, I tried to keep myself busy—anything to take my mind off the results. However, halfway through I noticed that, unlike the first IVF, my boobs were getting sore. I ignored it at first, but after a couple of days there was undoubtedly a definite change. I didn't tell Sam, as I didn't want to get his hopes up (or mine); so I just quietly made a mental note of this. We went for a walk a number of days before the test and I'm not sure what it was but I suddenly felt I was pregnant. It was a feeling I couldn't shake. I really wanted to shake it, because if I got hopeful, it would feel worse if I was wrong. But eventually I had to tell Sam, so two days before the test I told him that I think it might have worked.

"Really?" he asked.

"Yup. It just feels different this time. My boobs are sore, and I just have a feeling." I could tell that Sam wanted this to be true. That night, I prayed to anyone who would listen.

I guess I didn't pray hard enough.

The next day, I started bleeding. But this was not like anything I had ever experienced before. The pain was unbearable. I was sweating and rolling around on the floor. I lost count of how many times I had to change my sanitary towel. The blood was just seeping out of me. Sam was so sad about it obviously not working, but he was scared too as he had never seen me in this state before. He was going to call the ambulance at one point, as he could see how much blood I was losing. I ended up sitting on the toilet and just crying as the blood flowed.

I knew this wasn't a period. This was a very early miscarriage. At one point, I passed what I can only describe as the biggest clot I had ever seen. I don't know why, but I knew this was my baby. I don't think I had imagined it; I think I had actually conceived. I shut the bathroom door, flushed the toilet, locked the door, and collapsed inwards.

I came out about an hour later and could see that Sam had also been crying. This was one of the few times that we just sat quietly and hugged. There was nothing to say. I didn't bother going for the blood test the next day. I didn't see the point. They were quite insistent, but after I nearly bit their heads off, they backed off.

After a week, I decided I needed to go and see Sarah the Reiki Master. I couldn't get out of the fog I was feeling. The first IVF was a fact-finding mission and, although it was hard to hear that it had failed, I had felt that we would learn something that would make the second one work. That hadn't happened. IVF Number Two, in reality, was as dismal as the first one. Hence, my visit to Sarah. I needed some answers.

I told her it hadn't worked out and that I guess my interpretation of the "eight" had been wrong. She didn't say much except that she was sorry and hoped that all the work we had done would have helped. I was usually a chatty "patient," but I was in a dark place, so I just lay there and said nothing. She worked quietly on me for about half an hour and then said, "I just want to let you know that your body tried really hard to keep the baby, but it couldn't hold onto it."

I must admit I was a bit taken aback, as I hadn't actually mentioned the fact that I had thought I had been pregnant that time. I felt lighter when I left, but I still couldn't shake the feeling of hopelessness that was starting to win over my optimism. That was the last time I saw Sarah. She was great and in true Selby style, I had stuck with the energy work until the bitter end, but I still hadn't got a baby, so it was time to move on.

I am not sure though what exactly happened during that final session, because when I got home that night, something in me just crumbled.

I came in the house, looked at Sam, and started sobbing. I went into my bedroom at 5:00 p.m. and I cried like I had never cried before. It was as though everything I had been holding in over the years came out. At points, I didn't even think I was crying about the IVFs. It was my Dad's death; it was the sadness in my relationship; it was missing my family; and of course, this big gaping hole in my life that was seemingly impossible to fill! I sobbed so hard it felt like my body was trying to get rid of every hurt that it had ever experienced. At one point, Sam came in the room, as I think he was getting concerned, but I couldn't even talk to him; my sobs were so violent, I couldn't explain how sad I was feeling. He did what he thought would help and brought me a glass of wine. I think he was at a loss. Later, I had to smile, as it was the first time in my life (barring sickness and extreme fasting for weight loss) that I didn't even want a drink.

Even though parts of that night were a complete blur to me, there was a point when I said either aloud or in my head, "Okay, I give up. I am no longer going to fight for this, Universe. If this is going to happen, it's over to you, and I will be okay with what you decide. I have one more IVF left in me, and then I am done. If there is anything I need to know, you had better let me know now."

I don't remember falling asleep, but it must have been late, as I didn't hear Sam come into the bedroom. I suspect he was probably listening outside the door until he was sure I was asleep, as he probably wanted to avoid all conversation at that point. I think that night he realized how on edge I was and the toll this was taking on me. I woke up the next morning and looked in the mirror. I contemplated not going to work—my eyes were so puffy it looked like I had an eye infection. I really didn't know how I was going to explain this and had to come up with something. My explanation was that I had put an essential oil on my pillow and I had had a bad reaction to it. In retrospect, I think that was pretty creative.

I woke up that morning with two things I didn't expect. The first thought in my head was that I had to quit my job. It was crystal clear to me that that had to happen. The second thought was that I knew if my third and last IVF did not work, then Sam and I would need to end our relationship. This thought had always been there, because I knew how important children were to Sam; but for me now the decision was made.

Sam was understandably wary of me the next morning. I think he was just glad I had stopped crying. "How are you doing?"

"Good," I said, "But I need to talk to you about a few things. First, I have to quit my job. Don't ask me why, but I woke up this morning and I just know that is what I need to do. Secondly, Sam, I only have one more IVF left in me and if it doesn't work, then we need to separate. It's not because I don't love you; it's because you want a child and I can't give you one. I can't selfishly be with someone for the next however many years who will always feel something is missing. Last night, I am not sure what happened, but that was the saddest I have ever felt, and I was scared. Right now, I need to move forward. We have one last chance and I will do everything in my power to make it work; but we both have to face the reality, right now, that we have a very low chance of success."

Sam can drive me crazy and we were already teetering on the brink, but I will never forget his response.

"I trust you, if this is what you think we need to do, then I'm happy to go along with it. It'll be very tough on one salary; but we'll make it work. But I don't think that just because we can't have children, we would be better off apart. I don't agree and I want to stay with you."

I let the second part go. My mind was made up and I knew in the long-term it would be best if we went our separate ways. But that was something I would deal with when the time came.

Up to this point, my job had been a huge part of my life. Advertising is a stressful job; it's a creative business, and frankly these days, it is not always profitable. In any creative industry that is not selling widgets, making money can be challenging. Everyone always talks about the advertising world during the Eighties, because I think that was the decade of excess in all things—money was flowing, clients were spending, there were long alcoholic lunches, and overall, it sounded like a blast. I joined the advertising world in 1991, the start of the recession. Nowadays, the competition is fierce and dollars are scarce, so you have to be smarter, more agile, and more creative than ever before.

What the more competitive environment does produce, though, is a lot of people who are passionate, dedicated, and willing to push the limits further, to make a difference for their clients. As a work environment, advertising is one of the best. Every day, my clients and my team challenged me, and I challenged myself. I was often stressed, knackered, and completely overwhelmed, all at the same time. At my job, I had worked with some of the smartest people I'd ever met, and I learned more about myself than in any other position, so I do not regret one moment of the time I spent there.

I knew I had to leave, but it was going to be tough. I was anxious about talking to my bosses. I didn't want to let them down and I knew I also had to tell them what was going on in my life, so that they'd know why I was leaving. I liked them and owed them that.

It actually took me three months to finally get up the courage to discuss it. I went for a glass of wine with the company president and told her the whole story. She was great about it. The good news was that I had obviously managed to hold it all together publicly, as she had no idea about my last three years of struggle. I told her that I had one last IVF in me and had to give it my best shot. I didn't even know if the job was a factor in terms of my being able to conceive or not, but I didn't want to always wonder "what if," so I needed to do this.

She gave me a hug, asked me when was the latest I could stay. I told her three more months, and she genuinely wished me the best of luck. That was one of the hardest things I had to do. I walked away from something that I loved, from people I'd spent the last ten years or so of my life with, for something that I didn't even know would make a difference.

Sam could see how upset I was when I got home. He poured me a glass of wine and said he hoped that this would all be worth it. Yeah, no kidding!

I met my good friend Christine that night. This was the friend who loved going to psychics and had recommended Gabrielle. I actually think she is a little psychic herself, as she has a very strong intuition and can often, not predict, but sense when things are afoot. I told her I was off all psychics from now on as so far nothing had come to fruition.

"Oh. I was going to tell you something that I thought you would want to hear."

Great. How could I not want to know what that was?

"What is it?" I asked.

"Well, you know Gabrielle. I went to see her again, just for myself, but I did ask about you."

I remembered picking out the "mother card" and Gabrielle telling me it looked like I would have babies, but possibly through medical intervention. I now needed to know what she had said.

Christine obliged. "She said that she could definitely see you with a baby and that you would conceive before the June solstice. June 21st."

Well, this was good news and very date-specific, which for a psychic is unusual. But remembering the number "eight" experience, I wasn't holding out much hope. This gnawed at me for quite a while, so I thought I would put Gabrielle to the test. I booked another appointment with her to see if she would give me the same information.

I really did like this woman. She was so practical, for a psychic. I went on the pretence of finding out about my sister and getting general career information. I told Gabrielle that my sister's baby was "conceived" on March 10 and the due date was December 4. These dates were pretty significant to me; they had spooked me out a little bit—March 10 was our Dad's birthday and December 4 was the day he'd died, so I was very curious about this in general. I really don't know if I believe in reincarnation, but my belief is that I always need to be open, because not everything can be explained by science or faith. So I asked, "Is my sister's baby actually my Dad coming back?"

She laughed, then surprised me with, "No, it's not your Dad; it's your Dad's Dad. He's coming back to have some fun in this world, as he left quite early last time."

I'd never met my Granddad; he had died aged forty-four.

"What else do you want to know?"

I asked again if I was going to have a baby and, if so, what the timing would be.

"Turn over a card." Yet again, the "mother card" came up, the Empress, the same as the last time.

"Yes," she said, "you are and you will conceive by the end of June."

Whoooa! She had passed my test. She had told me the same information as she'd told my friend Christine; so of course, it must be true!

Funny really. I thought I was being super clever by testing her information, but I guess, if she was a good psychic, she had probably figured that out already! Either way, I was impressed and I couldn't stop that little flicker of hope starting to burn again in the pit of my stomach. I didn't tell Christine or Sam about this one. I didn't want to give too much hope to Sam; I didn't want him to see how much I had slipped down the desperation scale; also I couldn't face the lecture on, "Should we be spending our money on that?"

Also, I didn't really believe that it could be true. I had been down this path before and gotten hurt. The protective shell that I had started out with on this journey was now just a flimsy film, which I knew could tear at any moment. The question now was, "What could I do to increase my chances of success for IVF Number Three?"

IVF #2

Suppression drug: None—"IVF light"
Fertility drug: Puregon—only 9 days
Eggs: 7
Fertilized: 4
Grades: Slightly better than terrible: 8-cell, grade 3; 8-cell, grade 3; 8-cell, grade 3; and one ungraded.
Result: Possibly a very brief pregnancy, followed by another big fat negative.
Cost: $10,000 + more wine + energy sessions
Insanity scale: 7 out of 10—became obsessed by "ovary" meditation, communicated with dead people, quit well-paying job.
Relationship: 4 out of 10

Go Big or Go Home

We scheduled our follow-up appointment after IVF Number Two with Dr. T. I wasn't expecting much. At this point in my unfertile career, like most other unfertiles, I felt like I knew more, had researched more, and was as up to speed on my "medical" condition as anyone could be.

Dr. T. didn't disappoint. I think he was as frustrated as we were that the results weren't better, especially based on my initial tests.

He knew I was a realist and liked to be treated as such. I told him this was our last go, so was there anything, anything at all, we could learn from the first two that would help on this one? He really didn't think so. The old lady IVF protocol had been discussed with the team and they still felt this was the right route to go. Lead follicles are something they can't do too much about. It really depends on how one's body responds to the drugs. He felt they had done pretty well to get seven eggs, based on the way it had gone. I actually agreed with him; based on what I had read, this was pretty good. I told him I thought I had in fact conceived and explained the extreme pain, blood loss, and cramping that had occurred.

"You may be right from what you've said. So there is some good news, if that is in fact the case, an egg might have taken." I filled in the rest of the sentence for him, "But now there might be a problem with my holding on to a baby."

"That is a whole different set of issues, but as it was so early and we are not even sure you were pregnant, let's just focus on the first part. The other good news is that Sam didn't faint."

I laughed. Sam didn't.

"Are we missing anything?" I asked. "I know all the tests have come back great, but Dr. T., my gut tells me there is something that we are not addressing." I'm sure he must hear this from every couple he meets, as we all believe that if we just look hard enough, we might find something that will help.

Dr. T. has a great "bedside manner," i.e. how to keep the crazies in line! "There might be, but we've checked all the things that we know might have an impact on fertility. In ten years' time, there may be something else that comes to light, but as of now, we're not aware of it. There are lots of theories out there that may or may not be right, but none have been tested to the point where there is any conclusive evidence."

I understood his position—the medical world needs evidence. Unfertiles just need one story where it all works out well at the end.

"Do you think we are right to stop trying after this one?" I asked.

"You know, I can't answer that. It is your decision. But I don't think the results will get any better. You have an egg quality issue and the world of science right now has no conclusive answers on how to improve that over time."

I knew in my heart of hearts he was right. I was now thirty-nine and the statistical success graph was taking a severe nosedive.

We booked the IVF Number Three to start at the end of May. Driving home, Sam asked, "Would you really not consider doing this a fourth time if this does not work?"

"I can't go through this again, Sam. I need to move on."

His silence told me he wasn't quite there yet.

I am a firm believer in changing something if it is not working. That night, I wrote down a list of everything I had tried to improve my odds of having a baby:

- Acupuncture
- Chinese herbs
- Massage
- Meditation
- Psychic

- Energy worker
- Exercise
- Supplements
- Less alcohol
- Better diet
- Quit my job

There must be something I was missing or something everyone was missing. There was no way I was going to do this IVF without knowing that I had uncovered every stone and found the best people to help me crack this mystery.

I sat down and reviewed my list. What was I going to keep going with and what was I going to cross off my list? Back to Google. After emerging from the Google madness, I had a new list. A list that was going to get me a baby:

- Acupuncture: Try again.
- Chinese herbs: Reluctantly try again.
- Massage: Done with. I didn't really like massage and it was expensive.
- Meditation: On the fence. Likely will keep going.
- Psychic: I couldn't actually write this one down as Sam might find the list.
- Energy worker: Continue, but with a new person.
- Exercise: Continue.
- Supplements: Continue.
- Less alcohol: Arghhh! ... I suppose so ... but nearer the time of the IVF.
- Better diet: Continue.
- Job: Find something more flexible and with fewer hours.

Then my Google buddy identified some new candidates to try:

- Fertility Yoga
- Immune testing

- Couples counselling
- Reflexology
- Art

Thank goodness I had decided to quit my job; being unfertile is a full-time occupation. Mind you, I had agreed to work a further three months to ensure a smooth transition, so I was in fact still employed. Fitting all this in, even in the short-term, was going to be a challenge.

I like systems, so I started at the top of the list: Traditional Chinese Medicine. Although my previous experience had not gotten me the results I had wanted, there was too much evidence that this could really make a difference, so I couldn't ignore it. My sister swears to this day that she thinks it was instrumental in her success. She had continued with acupuncture throughout her entire pregnancy and finally, aged forty-two, Jane had given birth to a healthy, baby boy, Henry. So I felt I should really give Chinese Medicine another go. But I wasn't prepared to go down the same route as before. I looked at all the options out there and decided, really based on nothing, that the reason the acupuncture hadn't worked last time was because my doctor had not been Chinese.

A real, Chinese Chinese Doctor would make all the difference. I'm not sure how I could have overlooked this the last time, but now I was convinced this was the problem. I'm sure I don't need to point out the fallibility of my argument here!

The difficulty was that I didn't know any Chinese Chinese Doctors. And this was even more problematic, as I also decided that "real" Chinese doctors do not need to advertise. I mean if they're really good, aren't they always busy? This led to a bit of a dead end for a while and, because I didn't explain the reason why I was looking for a doctor, not many people could recommend one.

Just as I was coming to the conclusion that I would in fact have to resort to one of the advertised doctors, my luck changed. I met a girl at a dinner party who had had a tumour in her neck that had supposedly been diagnosed as cancerous. Rather than pursue the Western medical route, she had decided to try alternative medicine. She said she had been referred to an incredible Chinese doctor and was now cancer-free. Now, before you think that I am too naive, I knew there were probably a hundred reasons why she had beaten cancer, if in fact she had ever had cancer, as I didn't get all the facts. I didn't quiz her on this, quite simply because I didn't want to know. Time was not on my side and I had no better options, so he was my man. I got his address in Vancouver's Chinatown and set off.

I arrived at the address and was totally excited. This was the real deal. Shelves stacked with herbs and everyone in the store was Chinese. The only thing that perturbed me a bit was not seeing any signs for the doctor. I asked the assistant selling the herbs and she pointed to an old man sitting at a table at the back of the store and told me to join the queue. You don't make appointments; you just turn up and hope you get to see him. This is okay if you're not working, but when you have a day job, it makes it a little tricky. You can't just tell your boss or your clients that you're off to Chinatown to sort out your womb and you're not really sure when you'll be back. That day, I was lucky though. I was next in line, so one step closer to finding out what was wrong with me. I got a few funny looks from the other customers, as I'm sure they were all wondering what a Caucasian business chick was doing in a Chinese herb store. They didn't have to wait long to find out.

One thing I had not anticipated was that the doctor wouldn't know what "infertility" is. I mean he knew, but they call it something else in Chinese Medicine and his command of English was poor, though not as poor as my command of Chinese. So, in my wisdom, I thought, like many ignorant Caucasians, that if I shouted loudly enough he would understand me. Big mistake! I got so loud that all the people in the line now knew what my issue was, but, not only that, because the table was in the open, they also found out how regular my periods were, what the blood was like, why I wasn't married, and how long I had been an unfertile. But I didn't care, this chap was going to get me a baby and I loved him already. He must have been about ninety, had beautiful eyes, but most of all, he said those magic words, "We'll get you a baby!" At least, I think he said this; the language problems didn't help, but this is what I heard. He told me my kidneys were weak and that my mind was full. Again!

No kidding, when you're working full-time, are renovating (yes, for some inexplicable reason, Sam and I thought it would be good for the relationship to "take on a project" to bring us closer together. Just for the record, if you're thinking about doing this, don't), and going through infertility, no wonder your mind is full. I want to meet those people that have empty minds, as that seems to be the way to go. No doubt they are the ones with ten million kids and are the "earth mothers" of this world.

Another thing that proved a tad problematic was the herbs themselves. At the first clinic, all the herbs came in little pre-made bags that you just added to water. Here in Chinatown, I got the real herbs in all their glory. I listened to the instructions several times. They sounded simple enough: mix five cups of water with the herbs; boil down to one cup; add more water; boil down again to get two full doses. What they didn't tell me was that this process takes about two hours, and to make sure I would drink it in the morning I had to prepare it the night before. So after a long day at work, I'd come home and spend the evening cooking herbs that literally made the house reek. The tricky thing was that you had to get it just right to make sure you got the two full doses.

Many times, I couldn't see how much water I had put in and ended up sweating over the stove for two hours. I would end up with about a quarter of a cup of super-concentrated potion. I had to admit this was tough. It felt like a huge effort and again I wasn't exactly sure it was going to work. There was one time, I remember, when something pushed me over the edge. I was late home from work and couldn't make the drink at night. So I had to set my alarm to get up two hours earlier and make the drink in the morning. The house stank, I was knackered, and when I finally finished making the drink, it was so concentrated that I threw up. This was becoming exhausting. It is also worth mentioning that every time I visited the doctor, I came out with two plastic bags full of herbs that I would have to hide in my office until the end of the day and sneak out when most people had left, so they couldn't ask me what was in the bags.

Every week, I'd trudge back to the doctor and he'd tell me that my kidneys were getting stronger. Great, I'd say, and would purchase several more bags of the magic formula. I really trusted this chap. I think because he was really old, which I equated to being wise, he had the world's most peaceful smile, and I truly felt he could make me "normal" enough to conceive a child. In addition, he seemed very sure he could help me have a baby. To me, it was worth waiting in line every week just to hear those words. But all good things come to an end.

I went in one day and the woman told me that he was taking some time off. Something didn't feel right. Not only was I horrified that my Chinese "rock" was not around to tell me my kidneys were getting better, but I had a funny feeling she was covering something up. I asked when he was going to be back, but she didn't really answer and said, "Soon," and that I should keep going with the herbs until I could see him again. I told Sam that this didn't feel right and that I had an inkling that this doctor was not going to be around for too much longer. Sam was horrified, too. Not that he believes in anything alternative at all, but I think my faith in the doctor had rubbed off on him and he was starting to buy into the fact that the doctor could be our saviour.

It went from bad to worse. I called the shop every week and every time the woman would tell me that the doctor was okay, just relaxing as he had been a bit ill, but was now doing fine. Finally, he came back one day and I was elated. It was all going to be fine. I rushed down to see him and was totally relieved, because he looked the same, maybe a bit tired, but nothing too serious. However, I still had this nagging fear that he was not going to be with me for the whole journey. I am not sure if it was this, or the fact that I was finding it more and more difficult to keep the herbs down and make the friggin' drink. He said my kidneys were much stronger, but my womb was still a bit "cold," so we needed to work on that, as eggs do not like "cold" environments.

"Maybe we could try a hot water bottle instead of the herbs," I suggested hopefully. My sense of humour was lost on this chap.

I kept up with the medicine for a few more months, but the herb-making was getting me down. I was tired of cooking for hours every day. More often than not, the mixture I ended up with was either super-concentrated or too weak. Also, my body had started to reject it. Even the smell of the herbs was making me gag.

On my next visit, the doctor was absent again. After that, I called the shop a lot, as I was getting very concerned that I had not seen him in a long while and that maybe we needed to adjust the herbs. The woman was very vague about his whereabouts and just kept telling me he was resting and would be back soon. I was beginning to panic as my IVF was only a few months away at this point.

A couple of weeks later, when I had run out of herbs and couldn't make an appointment because he had not returned to work, I bumped into the girl who had cured her cancer; she told me that my Chinese doctor had died.

What the hell? I was devastated! Not just because he truly was a lovely man whom I thought was a very good soul, but also because a part of me was angry. Here I was on my last IVF, I thought I had found my saviour, and now he was dead. I mean, how good was he if he couldn't cure himself? He was meant to give me a child, not die on me.

Had I wasted my time for the last few months? I know I was being pretty selfish, but I felt like the rug had been pulled out from under me. The only positive thing to come out of this was that I could stop cooking the herbs. But, if I was still committed to this path, I had to find another Chinese doctor and fast.

Chinese Dr. number one—I had ruled out as incompetent.

Chinese Dr. number two—He had ruled himself out by dying. I was hoping three was my lucky number.

I actually found another one pretty quickly. Time meant that I couldn't follow my previous strategy of "waiting" for recommendations, so I scoured the internet for "specialists" in this field; and, by the way, my criteria of the doctor having to be Chinese was still very much in place. I finally found a doctor and his wife who ran a practice. They were a team. He diagnosed and recommended the herbs, and she did the acupuncture. I liked them straight away. Language was challenging again, but not quite as bad as before. But what swung it for me was that he said, "You can cook the herbs yourself, or we can do it for a fee of $10 a month." I loved this doctor! Little did he know that I probably would have paid a $100 a month not to cook those herbs! Every week, he gave me a 7 Up bottle filled with the evil liquid, which I dutifully took. My new trick was to hold my nose, so the smell didn't make me vomit before I could take it!

The acupuncture was different too. Previously, when I had had it, the needles were placed all over my body. It felt great, I must admit, but the results hadn't worked. This woman seemed more intuitive. She felt around my body and focused very much on my womb area. She kept saying, "Too cold, too cold—we have to warm you up."

After several minutes, either I was delusional, or something was actually happening. It is hard to explain, but I felt warm rushes of energy where the needles were; as if warm water was circulating in the areas where she was working, and my feet got hot. That never happens—my feet are usually in a state of permafrost.

I enjoyed working with this pair. Maybe because I felt they were focused on the issue at hand, but also because, at the back of my mind, the thought had lodged that perhaps I wasn't conceiving because I had a "cold womb." Again, it was probably complete nonsense, but at least it was something I could try to do, if nothing else.

The other thought that lodged in my brain after my hours of Googling was that my immune system might be at fault. My Mum had rheumatoid arthritis, which is an autoimmune disease, and through my research there were a few threads that seemed to link this to infertility. I asked Dr. T. about this. The clinic had done some initial screening on me and the results were negative for lupus/rheumatoid, etc., so he didn't think there was an issue. However, he did say that often with autoimmunity, it is very hard to get a positive read.

This bee in my bonnet would not go away, but there didn't seem to be any other way in Canada for doing more detailed testing or screening. In truth, it seemed most medical professionals I discussed it with didn't really buy into the idea that there may be a link between autoimmune issues and infertility. None of my results showed any conclusive reason to pursue it, so I felt as though I might have to abandon this theory.

Then one day, I was surfing online and found a clinic in the States. This was a topic they actually specialized in, conducting a really deep and detailed level of testing of the immune system. Essentially, the theory was that with some women their immune system may be on "high alert," meaning it would try to destroy any foreign bodies that entered the system. In this case, the system misinterprets an embryo as a foreign object or cancer cell, and hence the body attacks it.

The detailed information really did make my head hurt, but what caught my eye was that it felt very much geared to the group suffering from "unexplained" infertility. Their typical patient is 38.6 years (plus or minus two years), has been unsuccessful 4.4 times (plus or minus two), would be nearing the end of their reproductive years, and, more often than not, does not know why they can't conceive. Give or take a couple of statistics, this was basically me, so although it was a long shot, I thought it was worth digging into a bit more.

Before I contacted them though, I tried to research as much as I could about them; I was concerned that I had never heard of them before, so I was skeptical to say the least. I asked my family doctor about it and drew a blank. I called Dr. T. and he was actually aware of the clinic. He did not have any strong feelings either way about it, but did mention that there was definitely a split opinion about the clinic and their findings. Many in the medical profession thought it was a money-making scheme, but Dr. T. couldn't really say either way as he did not know enough about them and whether they had had enough success to warrant a look or not. However, at that time, my clinic did not follow the American clinic's theory.

Did I really want to go down this path? I, like Dr. T., had my reservations, and the testing looked complicated and long. Plus, the treatment seemed quite extreme. But, yet again, I had promised myself and Sam that after all this I had to walk away with the knowledge that I had done everything in my power to have a child.

So I called them to set up an initial consultation. They went through my family history and Sam's family history, our IVF history, and results and failures. Based on family history and all the information we shared, they suggested that I do the autoimmune blood test panel, as I looked like I had enough risk factors to warrant this. No surprises there.

I agreed to do all the blood tests and they also recommended that I do an endometrial biopsy to see if a certain type of lymphocyte—called a CD57+—were present in the uterine lining. To this day, I really don't know enough about the different tests, what they do, or what they really mean, but I knew these cells, if they are present, are not a good thing.

The trouble was that as I soon found out what was needed I couldn't get anyone to help me deliver the blood samples or do the biopsy. I went to my family doctor, as the clinic inferred that there would not be an issue with this because they had many people who came from Canada. Not so. My doctor did not understand the testing. It seemed that most of it was not being done in Canada, so she couldn't authorize the tests or recommend a lab to do them. Also she couldn't point me in the right direction—this was such a specialized field.

Mmmmm! Back to Google.

I found out that a few people were in a similar situation to me. I found a place in Toronto that could do it at the time, but nowhere in Vancouver. I asked the US clinic if they had any recommendations and if there were any other clinics in the States nearer the Canadian border, but I was not getting anywhere. I think today there are likely more options, but I was getting more and more frustrated.

I called Dr. T.

"Look," I told him, "I know that you don't buy into this as a cause for my infertility and I totally respect that, but can you help me get the blood tests and the biopsy done? I have tried every other avenue, Dr. T., and I keep hitting roadblocks. I wouldn't ask unless I was desperate. You know this is my last go-round and you know that I need to know I have done everything— please, please, please!" I added.

There was silence on the other end of the phone. Then he said, "Okay."

If I had been in the same room as Dr. T., I would have kissed him right there and then. I knew I had made the right choice of specialist. Not because we were getting fantastic results, which we weren't, but because he never once let his ego or his beliefs get in the way of trying to figure out why I couldn't get pregnant. I knew he didn't believe that this was likely to yield any results and that it would probably be a waste of time and money, but he seemed to understand better than most that I am the kind of person who needs to know I have tried everything before walking away.

There was a special way the tests had to be done within a set time. Dr. T. set it up for me and said he would do the biopsy. Everything had to be shipped overnight and labelled correctly, and the exact protocol had to be followed, otherwise we would have to repeat it. I knew asking him to do this a second time would be pushing my luck, so I made sure we had all the correct paperwork and information. The biopsy was relatively straightforward: just a quick scrape of the uterine lining, then drop the cells into a tube with the correct liquid, and ship them to the US.

When I walked into the lab for the blood tests, I was a little surprised to find a bed. I asked why and the nurse replied, "We think you'll need one. Either you will faint or your veins will collapse. We have to draw about sixteen vials of blood."

I saw Sam's face blanche. "Would you like the bed?" I joked. He stayed till about vial eight before he excused himself.

My veins held up. The nurses were amazed that I kept pumping blood; although I was definitely light-headed toward the end, it was nothing that an orange juice and muffin couldn't solve. The nurses were very systematic about labelling and ensuring they followed the instructions given. They were also curious about the testing, so I filled them in as much as I could in my layman's way and thanked them profusely. I knew this was outside the norm for them and they were indulging me, but they had been briefed that this was my last go-round so they were on my side.

A couple of days later, the US clinic called and let me know that the blood samples had arrived and it looked like they had been labelled correctly. However, the biopsy had not. I told them it had been done and shipped on the same day, so it should be there. I phoned my Canadian clinic and asked for the shipping information, as I knew the labels were correct. They gave me the information and I tracked it down to a customs office in the States. I asked them if it had left the office and they said yes.

"Are you sure, because no one has received it and it has human tissue in it and needs to be tested within a certain timeframe. Please, can you double check?"

I was dealing with a woman and I thought, if I explained why it was so important, she would prioritize helping me. It worked. She said, "It looks like it has left this office, but I will do one more look around for you."

A few minutes later, she came back to the phone. "I found it," she said. I think she was as pleased as I was. It's funny when you let people in a little bit and ask for their help, nine times out of ten, they don't disappoint.

She said, "It was such a small box, it had been missed. It was under the same shipping number as the blood test, but must have gotten left behind."

"Can you send it straight away?" I asked.

"No problem. I will do it now."

I thanked her, hung up, and rang the clinic. They said the sample should still be okay if they got it within twenty-four hours. They did. Who says customs people are unhelpful? That woman saved me from begging Dr. T. for a second time and having my poor uterine lining scraped again. Now, we just had to sit and wait for the results, the results that I hoped would contain the answer and get me a baby.

I was meeting Debbie—the friend who had decided to use a sperm bank—that weekend; we were going to go for a run together. It had been a while since I had seen her, so I was interested to see how things had been going with her and if she had decided when she was going to inject the sperm that she had put on ice at the clinic. I had let her into my world of IVF a bit, as she was a close friend and I felt that it was the right thing to do.

As we were running, I asked if she had decided on a date. She told me she had injected the donor sperm already and would find out in a couple of weeks whether it had worked.

"Wow!" I said, "What did you have to do?"

She said it was pretty much the same process as with Chris, her gay-guy-donor. She had to monitor herself closely, with the clinic helping this time, and when she was ready to ovulate, she had to go to the clinic and have the defrosted sample injected.

"How was it?"

"Pretty painless," she said. But the bad news was that her chances of success were pretty low too, based on her age, the same as anyone doing it naturally, which they said was about fifteen to twenty percent.

"Well, good luck," I said, "and fingers crossed." I suddenly asked, "Should you be running? Could it drop out?"

She laughed. "I don't think so. The clinic okayed that I could run and I can't lie in bed all day. Most women have no clue they're pregnant until they miss their first period, so I'm just carrying on as normal."

I admired her for that. I think I would have gone to bed and not moved.

I didn't hear from Debbie and after two-and-a-half weeks, I left her a message. I figured that she hadn't called me, because it had worked and she didn't want to upset me.

"Look, Debs," I left her a message on her phone, "I think the reason you've not called me is because you're pregnant. Despite my emotional fragility and my unexplained inability to conceive, you can still share your good news with me. If it is in fact true, I am super pleased for you. You have not had it easy, so don't be an arse; call me!"

She called. My message had worked and so had the injection of sperm. Debbie was pregnant! I was truly glad. She had not chosen an easy path and she was going to need all the support she could get; she was still with her partner who was lukewarm—to say the least—on the idea of having a baby.

So now, out of six friends, four were pregnant. I thought that deserved a nice bottle of Pinot Grigio.

I got a call from the US clinic to set up a review of my results. We arranged for a conference call with the doctor. We read our copy of the results as he went through them. It was very complicated. I took as many notes and asked as many questions as I could, but it was hard to keep track. Overall, my system did seem to be in immune-overdrive, which they felt was affecting my chances of conceiving. In fact, they said that they really didn't expect me to conceive with results like mine. The good news was that I did not have "killer" cells in the uterine biopsy. So, although my body was hostile, my womb, if we could get everything else under control, did not have the evil embryo killers in there.

A couple of things struck me as we went through the results. One was that I had heterozygous MTHFR gene. This is essentially a mutation of a certain gene, not particularly relevant to infertility, but there is a theory that if you have this mutation it often means that you cannot absorb vitamins properly—vitamins like folic acid and some of the B complex. Some people in the medical community think this can lead to heart disease, stroke, and many other disorders, including an increase in autoimmune diseases. This in fact made sense to me as my father's side of the family was riddled with heart disease and my Mum had rheumatoid arthritis. They also tested—I found this fascinating—whether genetically I was too similar to my partner. Apparently, if you are too similar, it can be a problem. I got rather lost in many parts of the results, so at some point with all the various names of cells, tests, and results, my brain seemed to shut down.

In the end, they concluded, much like the rest of the doctors out there, that my chances were less than ten percent for conceiving without any treatment and no guarantees with treatment. I asked them what treatment they recommended, holding my breath, as I knew that what was coming would be expensive.

At the very basic level, they recommended taking a mix of vitamins and a baby aspirin, every day of my life from now onwards. This was for the MTHFR gene issue, because in their opinion addressing this was important for my general health, as well as for any infertility issues. I was not quite prepared for the next bit. They recommended that I undergo a therapy they called LIT. I've compiled this description from several online sites: "*Lymphocyte Immunization Therapy or LIT is a procedure whereby white blood cells from the prospective father are injected into the skin of the prospective mother to prepare the maternal immune system for pregnancy.*" Bottom line is it should stop the mother's body from attacking any foreign tissue from the father, as far as I could make out.

I asked what this would involve and found out that the procedure has not actually been performed in the States since 2002, by FDA ruling. The clinic, however, believed in its effectiveness and had set up another clinic to carry out the procedure—in Mexico. Holy Moly! The treatment itself sounded scary enough and travelling to the US would have already put a financial strain on us; but having to go to Mexico suddenly put this into a whole different league.

The other treatment the clinic recommended involved a product that contains an antibody extracted from the plasma of over a thousand donors to be intravenously injected into the woman's bloodstream!

We sat and listened, tried to ask the right questions, and made as many notes as we could, so we would know everything that was involved. In retrospect, I think I absorbed only about twenty percent of the information. The next step for us was to think about treatment and then get started. We thanked the doctor, made sure the line was dead, and looked at each other.

"Bloody hell, Sam," I said, "This is pretty hard core. If we do this, we will have to remortgage the apartment."

"What do you think?" he asked.

"Honestly, I don't know at this point. There's a part of me that believes my immune system or some part of my system is out of line, so in theory this makes sense in terms of a possible reason why we can't conceive. But, no offence, do I really want your blood cells and the plasma of over a thousand people injected into my body through a procedure that is not even approved in the States? I wish I had the knowledge or brains to understand it all, but I can't. I feel I would need to become an expert immunologist to even start comprehending whether this makes sense. But then the unfertile voice is telling me, 'What if this is it?' Can we go for a drink to discuss and compare notes?"

"I thought you weren't drinking so much before the IVF."

"Oh, for fuck's sake, give me a break. I'm in the midst of making a decision about whether to hop on a plane to Mexico to undertake a procedure that is not even allowed in the States and which involves other people's bodily fluids, and you are making me feel bad about having a bloody glass of wine. Don't bother. I'll work it out on my own."

I stormed off, found a nice little bar, ordered a glass of Pinot Grigio (my IVF wine of choice), and didn't even look at the pile of test results and notes I had brought with me. This was a turning point for me. I felt the universe was pushing me to see how far I would really go to get this baby. Despite the fact that I had sworn to the world that it was over after this try, whether it worked out or not, I was a true unfertile inside and couldn't quite stop myself from pushing for every possible solution. But, I decided the insanity had to stop. Although I actually thought there was something in this and had read that the clinic had had many successes, I knew that I was not going to pursue this route. It felt too extreme, even for me. If guarantees were involved, that would be different, but everyone has a line I think, and suddenly I had found my line. If this was what I was going to have to do to get a baby, then I would not be getting a baby.

I went home and found Sam reading the information. "Make any sense?" I asked.

"Not really," he replied. "Did it make sense to you?"

"I didn't actually read it," I confessed, "but I don't want to do it."

"Why not?"

"I'm not sure. I've been prepared to do a lot of things to get this child, but for me this just crosses my line. I never even thought I had a line, but it appears I do."

I was waiting for him to convince me otherwise, but he didn't.

"Good. I don't want to either. I mean, can you imagine how many needles would be involved?"

I laughed. I knew it was more than that, but I was relieved. Sometimes, Sam surprises me.

I sent a copy of the results to my clinic. Dr. T. read them and asked me what I was going to do. I said I would take the vitamin suggestions, folic acid, and baby aspirin. I told him I couldn't do the others. So, it was on to Plan C or whatever plan we were on by now.

Art and Love

That night I looked at my list again. Fertility yoga was up next. Back to Google. I found a yoga clinic that was not too far away and signed myself up for the six-week fertility yoga class.

I was a bit apprehensive attending the first class, because I was not really sure what this yoga entailed. I was secretly dreading that there would be a lot of "sharing." It didn't disappoint. I walked in and everyone was sitting in a circle. Oh God! I nearly bolted for the door, but it was too late. The teacher had introduced herself and me to the group. I don't know why I was so averse to sharing, considering I am now telling everyone my whole story in this book! I think it is the "group sharing" that I am not very good at.

The class started. It was my worst nightmare. Everyone told a little bit of their story and about where they were in their infertility journey. I had the same feeling that I had had in the clinic originally. I didn't want to be there; I didn't want to be part of this group; and sharing would make it all the more real. Plus, it was very depressing. I was depressed enough. I felt sorry enough for myself and now I had to feel sorry for everyone else. I struggle with hugs too.

Then the teacher announced that she too was an unfertile and was trying to conceive. Whoooa! Hang on a minute! How do you know this stuff actually works if you haven't managed to conceive? I'm here to find something that works, not something that just feels good.

One woman started crying while she was sharing. Her story was sad and I didn't blame her for feeling like she did. That was how I felt most of the time. But I wanted to hear from people that it had worked for, not from those in the same position as me.

Anyway, I had paid, so I might as well give it my best shot. As

I was lying on the floor with my hips resting on a bolster and my legs up against the wall "to help blood flow," I just got angry. Why do I have to do this? It sucks. I did find out that my hips are incredibly tight. The hip openers have always been a struggle for me; it can actually be excruciating at some points. I literally seize up after holding a position for a while, and occasionally when I stand up, one of my legs is "dead," so this can result in a lot of instability—physically, not emotionally!

Actually, the class itself was fine and relaxing. I did feel "warmer" afterwards, but I couldn't shake off the sadness. I didn't know if I could handle another five weeks of feeling this every Wednesday night. I needed some encouragement and hope at this point, not tears and hopelessness. Over the coming weeks, the teacher noticed I was quieter than most in the class and asked if everything was alright. I told her I liked the stretches, but that I found it a bit depressing as everyone in the class was trying to have a baby and none of us had succeeded. As I've said, I'm not a sharer, so I found the "circle time" a bit stressful. She told me she did private classes if that was something I wanted to consider.

As I was leaving, she also said, "You know your right hip is extremely tight and often that is because you are not letting your female energy flow. I can feel it every time you walk by me." I had not mentioned my hip, so I was a little surprised by her comment.

I phoned Maxine that week.

"How's it going?" she asked. I told her about my new list, which number I was on, and the whole autoimmune saga.

"Jeez!" she said. "I can't believe the Chinese doctor died on you!"

"I know—of all the things—that was the one that got me too. How's chemo?"

"Pretty shitty. I've lost all my hair now and it's quite surprising how large my head is under all those fake blonde tresses. I had to buy a wig for work, which, by the end of the day, is so itchy I want to scratch my head off."

I told her about my yoga classes and my inability to share. "I'm just getting sick of being an unfertile, Maxine. It's draining and bloody expensive."

"Try having cancer," she said.

"Why do you always have to play that card? You know I can't beat that."

"I know," she said, and laughed. "What's next on your list?"

"Well, I was reading somewhere that if you're aligned with your passion, then your body is happy and may help you conceive."

"I don't think you should become a sommelier," she said. "That definitely won't help."

Funny lady.

"No," I told her. "I was going to go to a fine arts school when I was younger and I was thinking I should get back into art, because I used to love it; although I'm not very good, I could lose myself for hours just painting and drawing. So I signed up for a life drawing class."

"Is that the one with naked bodies?" she asked.

"Yup," I responded.

"You know you're clutching at straws now," she said.

"Yup."

"Let me know how it goes."

I was pretty nervous turning up to class. It had been twenty years since I had last done any serious drawing and I had no idea what to expect. I walked into the class and there were about twelve of us. I noticed one guy straight away. He was gorgeous and talking to the woman next to me. Seriously, this chap was impressive. Since being with Sam, I had not really checked out too many guys, but I won't deny it had been a rough few years and I had that niggle in my head that we wouldn't be together if this last try didn't work. And having this piece of raw manliness next to me was distracting, to say the least.

I couldn't believe it when he came over to me and said, "You're one of the most attractive women I've met in a long time."

Sorry, that was my inside voice. He didn't even notice me. Imagine my surprise when he stood up and declared he was the teacher. This couldn't get any better, a ripped, drop-dead gorgeous guy who had talent. This was going to be the best art class ever!

The class was good, but tough. I was very rusty and became frustrated. The model was an old man and we all sat around him in a circle with our easels. The good news was that we didn't have to share and this was the first group I had been in for a while that had nothing to do with infertility. The bad news was that I had the unenviable position of being directly in front of the model, so my "scene" was full-frontal willy on display. I had wondered why that was the only chair free! My classmates had obviously done this before. I really appreciate those models, not only are they brave enough to get naked in front of strangers, but they're totally comfortable with their bodies, and have the patience to sit there for a couple of hours. Yet, trying to accurately represent a seventy-year-old willy was a challenge. It didn't help that every time the teacher came over, I blushed like a schoolgirl.

But I did love the class. I realized art had been out of my life for a long time and even if this would, as I suspected, have no impact whatsoever on my ability to conceive, by being so engrossed in something, I forgot for a short time that I couldn't seem to have a child. For me, this was worth it.

I couldn't help but tell Sam that I had the most attractive art teacher ever. He was nonplussed, but I had to explain why every Saturday afternoon my hair was done and my lipstick was on. The art teacher brought his girlfriend to the next class. She was equally as attractive as he was. Funny that.

The three hours passed very quickly.

There was one girl who was not only brilliantly talented, I thought, but happened to be beautiful too. I noticed each week that the teacher paid special attention to her and I had a feeling he was interested in more than her art. I had, at this point, gotten over the fact that someone ten years his senior and at least ten pounds heavier was probably not going to make it into his radar. I had the sense that something was burgeoning between these two.

The next class, he announced publicly that he had broken up with his girlfriend. My inner voice told me that next he was going to say (publicly still) that there was someone in this art class who had turned his world upside down and that he could no longer keep it a secret. Yay, my life was about to change forever. I didn't think I should mention the small issue of infertility at this point in our relationship. I waited, but nothing came.

I noticed at the end of the class that he and "Miss Talented and Beautiful" went for coffee. My gut had been right again. I told Sam I had broken up with the art teacher and was back with him, if he was willing to take me back.

"I didn't realize you had left me," he said. "Only in my head," I replied.

I took a couple of classes with the teacher over the next few months and I worked really hard at my art. It did take my mind off all the other stuff that was going on in my world. Most of the people in that class were actually art students or in the art world already, so they were much better than me, but I tried. I remember in the last class when, guess what, teacher and "Miss Talented and Beautiful" made their romance public, he came over to me and this other guy, Andrew (who were the only two "non-artists" in the class), and said, "When you two joined, I didn't think you had much talent, but I was wrong; you've come a long way. Keep it up."

Yay! Andrew and I gave each other a high five, even though I realized it was a back-handed compliment. We knew we were the worst in class, but we hadn't given up and actually had gotten better over the weeks. We had finally been accepted into the group and this was one group I didn't mind being part of. No sharing, no tears, just drawing, and wine and cheese. I loved it.

I didn't sign up for the next class since the IVF was approaching. I felt that all my energies should be focused on that. Plus, we had no money to pay for it, but I knew one day I would go back to art classes.

Going into this last IVF, Sam and I were struggling. Maybe it was because we had gone through three years of disappointment; maybe because we still didn't know the reason why we couldn't get pregnant; or maybe it was the fact that we were approaching the last IVF. We had always been a "quiet" kind of couple—neither of us are chatterers—but we had become even more distant over the last few years. Whatever the reason, I felt we needed to do something. Not only was the infertility a big issue, but we are very different people. Sam loves order, planning, and tidiness. I am a bit chaotic and untidy. Just living together makes this challenging, let alone having the added stress of trying for a baby. I had previously suggested counselling to Sam, as I thought having a third party involved might help us work through some of our issues, because we didn't seem to be doing very well on our own.

Sam had not been interested before; he felt that we could sort it out ourselves. But things had changed for him too, and when I raised it this time, he agreed. He said that some counsellors were covered under his work plan and we should probably try that first. It made sense to me, so he said he would look into it.

I am not really sure what I expected from the session. The counsellor was very nice, but unfortunately, I felt she fell into the stereotypical image I had in my head: slightly hippyish, kind of fuzzy around the edges, and I got a sense that she was struggling with more issues than we were. So we did not get off to a great start.

She asked us why we were there. I didn't know where to start so I just launched in.

"Because we're going through IVF, we seem to be drifting apart, and we're fighting all the time. At times, I think I would be happier on my own."

Sam looked at me.

I should have shut up, but I couldn't stop myself. "I know it's important to be tidy, but occasionally I would love you to talk about world peace or even an item you see on the news versus, 'When did we last wash the sheets?' Conversation engages me emotionally and then I want to have sex. But the mundane stuff that fills way too much of our lives is already spilling over into our conversations and it's killing me. We can't talk about IVF, it's too depressing; housework is equally depressing to me, and you don't seem to be interested in anything else right now."

Sam just continued to look at me.

The counsellor decided it was time to join in. I wished she hadn't, as the first line out of her mouth was, "How does that make you feel, Sam?"

Really? That cliché? I know there's probably a good reason for working out how you feel, but I was just hoping for something more original. Sam ignored her question entirely and launched into his attack on me.

"For the record, I just like the house tidy because it's less stressful for me. I grew up with parents who constantly tidied up; so I've never been comfortable with mess and I don't understand why you can't just put your bloody clothes away instead of leaving them on the floor for a week. And when was the last time you initiated a conversation? Most of the time, you're online searching for a 'cure' for something that even the medical community can't explain, but you think you'll come up with the answer. I feel if I talk to you about so many things you'll bite my head off, so I just keep quiet."

Mmmmm! Well, that stung, but I knew it was true. I felt like it had been a stalemate for a long time. Until we could move on from this infertility issue, we didn't even know what was left for us to figure out, even if we wanted to be together and be happy. Maybe at this point we were one of those couples who thought a baby would "fix" them. I see how that can happen and how you end up telling yourself that your own misery is because you can't have a baby, and that once you get one, it will all become good again. But so far, this journey had just made the cracks bigger and I wasn't sure anything was fixable.

The counsellor, I felt, was next to useless. So far she had just asked a few standard questions that I felt were read off a sheet. I asked her directly if she thought we were in serious trouble as a couple. She announced that she didn't feel we were in any position to make a decision based on what we were going through. I said, "I know, but you must have seen hundreds of couples and, based on their interactions, don't you have a sense? My biggest fear is what if the next IVF works and we bring a child into a relationship that is gasping for its last breath? Shouldn't we know that sooner rather than later?"

"Well, ideally, yes," she said. "But I think we need to do some more work to determine that."

I asked Sam what he thought as we headed to the car.

He said, "Well, I could tell you weren't impressed."

"No, I wasn't Sam. I'm so fucking scared right now about everything: the last IVF, the fact that we seem to be miserable with each other. I just want to make sure that we want this baby for the right reasons and that we're going to be good enough parents for it. If we're fighting all the time, or worse, not even communicating, the poor kid will wish he'd stayed inside the Petri dish. Personally, all that hour with the counsellor did was get me more stressed. That woman is not going to help us figure anything out, in my opinion."

"Well, the good news is we were only covered for one session," Sam laughed.

I laughed too. "Was it me or was she terrible?"

"She was terrible," he agreed.

I can't claim that in the following months we resolved anything in our relationship, but I think we both knew the seriousness of what was at stake and started to make an effort on trying to focus on the positive attributes we each brought to the relationship. Some days, there weren't any, but sometimes there were. I also started to pick my clothes up off the floor. Sam, I noticed, started asking my opinion on news items or anything he had read recently. Not world peace, but the truth was that was probably over my head anyway.

The Last Kick at the Can

IVF Number Three was getting closer and I was getting more desperate. So desperate in fact that my next purchase was the video called, *The Secret*. A close friend recommended it to me, so I thought I'd give it a go. I don't know if many of you have read *The Secret*, but the essence of it is that if you have images of the life you want and view them every day, then subconsciously your mind will start to focus on the images, and slowly, but surely, they will materialize.

The first step is to create a vision board that contains images of the life you would like to lead. Put it somewhere where you can see it every day, take a look, and things will start happening.

Simple enough. I started gathering magazines and putting sticky notes on the pictures that I thought I would want my life to look like in the next few years. No surprises, I wanted to look like a pregnant woman, so I scoured the magazines and internet to find the perfect representation of a pregnant me! This didn't take too long. I found a fit, youthful, very pregnant woman who looked radiant. That was me. I cut it out and posted it on my vision board.

Sam saw this and said, "Who's that? She looks hot."

"It's me, pregnant, of course."

"Julie, it's called *The Secret*, not the 'Bloody Miracle Worker.'"

You can imagine my reply.

I found vision boarding quite fun; it helped me focus on what I wanted. For the record, my vision board had a pregnant woman, a beautiful home by the sea in Vancouver, a stately Georgian home in England, a very fit and relaxed picture of a yoga instructor, lots of dollar bills, and books. You might as well aim high if you're going to take the trouble to do this.

The challenge came when I had to choose which baby to put on the board. There are so many cute baby pictures to choose from, finding "my" baby was not easy. There were several contenders, but I settled on this little chap who had the most beautiful, big, blue eyes and looked like he would have a wicked sense of humour. In retrospect, I'm not sure why he had blue eyes; neither Sam nor I have blue eyes. It was his cheeky, knowing look that sealed it for me. Up he went on the board, on the back of the bedroom door, surrounded by images of my future, opulent life. Now, all I had to do was take a few seconds each morning, look at my board, and, wham, the universe would align, and I would have a baby.

I made Sam watch *The Secret* too. I could tell he didn't buy into it, but he didn't have any better ideas. A few weeks went by and Sam still hadn't done his vision board and it started to bug me. Since finding out that I had the infertility issue, I had started to feel pretty alone on this journey. The hard truth was that there really wasn't anything Sam could do and I think that must have made him feel pretty hopeless too. But considering I was reading, and desperately seeking the "cure," I thought it really wasn't too much to ask him to do a vision board.

After one particularly tough day, I lost it with Sam. It truly had nothing to do with him; I was just tired of trying, tired of holding it together, and wanted someone to blame. Sam just happened to be in the wrong place at the wrong time.

Me: "I guess you don't want a baby, then?"

Sam: "What are you talking about?"

Me: "I spend every spare minute I can trying something, anything, to get us a baby, and you can't even be bothered to do a bloody vision board. Is it too much to ask? It's just one thing. I'm running out of ideas and, yes, this is a pretty desperate theory, but nothing else has worked. I would really appreciate some support in whatever form you can muster up; but your vision board would be a good starting point."

Sam: "You really are incredible, Julie. You think you're the only one suffering in all of this. You have no clue what it feels like to not be able to do anything to help and make this happen for us. I have to sit by and watch you try everything, with no results so far, and it breaks my heart. So, stop being such a martyr. It's not my fault that things are the way they are, so stop blaming me. I'm doing my best and I'm sorry it's not good enough for you."

He then reached into his bag and threw his vision board at me and walked out.

I knew I had gone too far. Sam very rarely showed me his pain, but I could see how much he was hurting. I picked up his board and took a look. He had obviously put a lot of thought into it, which made me feel even worse.

Bugger! Why couldn't I have just kept my mouth shut and let him show me? My timing was awful.

Sam also had a very cute baby on his board, very different from mine—a more serious, intense child. He too had a few properties in beautiful places—Vancouver, South America, and there was generally a happy calmness to his board. I placed his board next to mine. They were not that dissimilar.

I left a note at the top of the stairs that he would see when he came in. "Sorry," was all it said. He ignored me as he got into bed.

I couldn't sleep and lay awake most of the night thinking how far apart we now were and how big the third party wedged between us had grown. Even if we did manage to have a baby, would we ever get back to how it was before? Some days I just didn't think so.

But as I lay there, I knew this train of thought would just take me even further down the dark hole I was in, so I tried to focus on what my next steps should be. I still wanted to continue the energy work, but needed to find someone new. So the next morning I started researching my next "person who was going to get me a baby." I eventually settled on a woman who lives on First Nations reserve land. I turned up as open-minded as always. One thing this journey has taught me is that I had a large capacity for delving into the alternative world.

Again, like the first energy worker, this woman had an amazing glow about her, a calmness and a surety of which I am always envious and slightly in awe. She lit some sage, "cleared" the room of negative energy, and began to work on me. Interestingly, as I returned for further sessions, the same little girl from my Reiki sessions came up time and time again. The good news was that she seemed happier and more excited to see me each time she popped into my head. She would take me on walks around her "hood," where there were beautiful fields and meadows. Overall, a pretty great time was had by all. I couldn't imagine who wouldn't enjoy these sessions! I would walk in tired, stressed, and anxious, and come out relaxed, calm, and feeling happy.

I asked her after a couple of sessions, "Are there any clues as to why I can't conceive?"

"I think you will conceive, but it feels like your body is fighting it for some reason. When I work on you, I get the image of a goalie who keeps batting away the pucks, and that's what it feels like to me: that something is mentally guarding your womb, but I am not sure why. My gut says it could be a past trauma that your body is trying to protect you from."

I told her about my past-life experience and the memory of a husband aborting a fetus from me. I also described the experience of the last IVF, during which I was sure I had been pregnant. So I asked her whether she thought maybe my body was protecting me from going through that again.

"I don't really need to know what it is," she said. "I am just going to focus on shifting this energy."

Incredibly, over the next few sessions, she started to work specifically on my womb area and I felt my whole body heat up. Whether it was my imagination or just me telling myself that was what was happening, my legs and lower regions would feel warm and tingly whenever I left. One day, before we were ready to start the IVF, she said, "I think the goalie is ready to leave."

About time! I was going in for my pre-IVF tests the next week.

I went into the clinic lab the next week to get the usual battery of tests. It was hard to describe how I felt. I was anxious and scared. There was an unspoken tension both in me, Sam, and, I think, the staff at the clinic, too. The staff, as always, were amazing, but it was different this time. They carried out the tests as normal, but there was that extra sense of finality as they wished me good luck again. I had built up a relationship with these people over the years and it was all going to come to an end, one way or another.

Dr. T. called me with the test results a few days later. No surprises. All was stellar again on paper. I was yet again the perfect candidate.

I had also asked Dr. T. to test my thyroid. I could not shake the feeling that my TSH levels were too high, indicating my thyroid gland was underactive. I had been reading even more about this and I couldn't understand why Canada's range was so much wider than the rest of the world's. The European literature I had read strongly advocated that anything above 2.5 was an issue for trying to conceive. My TSH was 4.8. I called Dr. T. back a couple of days later.

"Dr. T., I don't want to go into this IVF with a TSH reading this high. Don't ask me why, but I think this has something to do with why I can't get pregnant. I just can't get my head around the fact that the rest of the world views this differently from Canada. What can we do about it?"

"Well, we can always put you on medication to boost your thyroid, if you feel that strongly. It will take a while to get into your blood stream, so we can delay the IVF for a few weeks until your thyroid adjusts."

I hate taking any sort of medication, especially long-term medications like Synthroid, but I felt that if an underactive thyroid was possibly impacting my chances of getting pregnant, then I needed to do something about it.

"Yes. I want to start the medication."

"Okay," said Dr. T. "I'll write you a prescription and we'll get started on it."

Six weeks later, my thyroid reading was 2.19; acceptable by European standards. Going into my last IVF, I was on my B vitamin mix, baby aspirin, and Synthroid. Oh, and a warm womb from all the energy work! I felt I had done as much as I could; so now it was over to fate.

My Day Three tests were fine, so I was due to start the IVF old-lady protocol the next day. They put me on 200 IU of Puregon. A few days after the medication started, I went in for the usual blood tests. My reading was strong again. This time my E2 on Day Five was 1291. So, as with IVF Number Two, it was either lots of eggs or the dreaded scenario of lead follicles taking over again.

The clinic wanted to do the ultrasound on Day Seven.

I felt sick going in for the first ultrasound. My E2 count was at 3136. I no longer felt any kind of excitement, just dread. It was Dr. T. who was on front-bottom duties that morning.

"How are you doing?" he asked.

"Pretty nervous," I said, "But it will be what it will be, and I can't do any more so let's get on with it."

Shit. Shit. Shit. It was not good. My right ovary looked like it had another lead follicle with one already over 15 mm and two at between 10 mm and 14mm, and once again there were a few under 9 mm. My left ovary this time also looked like it had a lead follicle. It too had one over 15 mm and eight under 9 mm.

"Okay, let's see how the other eggs are coming along in a few days," he said, "and then we can make a decision."

"What decision?" I asked.

"Whether we should cancel. This is your last IVF, so I think if it's going badly we should stop. You can save some of your money and then try again later."

I had not thought about this as an option. I tend to be an all-or-nothing kind of person, but I did appreciate the fact that he was thinking of both saving us money and not wasting this last chance.

I called Sam and told him the news. I could tell by the silence he was really disappointed. I let him know that Dr. T. suggested that we could cancel if it didn't get any better. Sam was quite supportive of this, as he secretly didn't want me to stop after this go; but I was on the fence.

Two days later, I went back in for the ultrasound. I was prepared for what was to come. The lead follicles were getting bigger, but in my right ovary, five were now in the 10 mm to 14 mm range. In my left, the lead one was still growing faster and the others were just not catching up at a good rate. It was not Dr. T. who carried out the ultrasound this time, but the doctor said he would let him know the results. It was Saturday afternoon when Dr. T. called. I was sitting on the sofa, in my sweat pants, dreading the call.

"Julie?"

"Yup, it's me."

"I think we should cancel. It just doesn't look like the small eggs are going to catch up in time. We can increase the Puregon dosage a bit, but I just feel that this is not going to work out any better than the first two. So, bearing in mind the money and the fact that you have said you only have one more IVF in you, we should stop here."

I sat there for what seemed like ages, just not saying anything. I was upset and angry at the world and was all out of ideas.

Then I opened my mouth and said, "Nope. We're going ahead, Dr. T. This is my last IVF and, come what may, I want to see it through to the end. What I need you to do is to get me as many eggs as possible in the time we have. I know you do this every time, but don't worry about me. Just tell me when you think is the best time for retrieval."

"Are you sure?"

"Yes."

"Okay. I will see you every day from now on and I'll do my best to maximize what we can get."

"Thanks."

That is all he could do at this point.

I got off the phone and Sam was looking at me. "Don't you

think we should have discussed this, Julie, before you decided that we were going ahead? This is a joint decision and I'm pretty pissed off that you left me out of it."

He was right, of course. I should have asked. I didn't really have any excuses or solid reasons. I just said, "Sam, I'm sorry I didn't ask you, but I don't think you would have changed my mind. It's partly the fact that I just feel we should keep going, and partly based on the fact that I can't do this again, so it just felt like the only choice."

"Okay," he said. "But stop thinking this is just your journey— it's mine too."

I went for an ultrasound the next day. The lead follicles were big, but the little ones were catching up.

Dr. T. said, "We might lose the big ones, but I think we have to keep working for another day with the smaller ones. They're starting to catch up. It's a bit risky, but let's give it one more day."

The next day my E2 was at 13,050 and my final ultrasound showed I had five eggs over 15 mm and six between 10 mm and 14 mm. It was a long shot, but Dr. T. decided it was time for the Ovidrel.

"We've already gone on longer than I would like to. The lead ones are possibly overcooked, so yes, it's time. I think though we will only get about the same number as last time, but we may get lucky."

"Okay. So when should I come in?"

"Day after tomorrow," he said.

I told Sam what Dr. T. said we could expect. He didn't say much. I think because it was no better than last time, he probably thought we should have cancelled; but I appreciated his not saying it.

We had to do the "mother lode" Ovidrel shot that day.

I was amazingly calm during retrieval. I still found the process very painful and they loaded me up with drugs to help. This time, I put on my iPod and shut the world out. I didn't want to talk to Sam, the doctor, or anyone else. I just wanted to listen to music that made me forget everything (although not easy, when someone is twisting your ovaries around to try and find that magic egg that was going to give you a baby).

I noticed it was taking a while and I had to have quite a few doses of the happy drug to keep the pain at bay. I got the tap on the shoulder letting me know it was over and I took my earphones out. They said I should rest up a bit in the recovery room, because my ovaries had had a pretty rough ride.

We were both very quiet in the room. This entire IVF Number Three had a sense of finality about it from the get-go, and I think Sam and I were both so emotionally exhausted from the last four years that there really was nothing to say. The first time it was exciting; the second time soul-destroying; this last time, I was just numb.

I noticed Dr. T. coming into the room. This was unusual, as he had never popped by before. I assumed it was because this was the last one and maybe this would be the last time I would see him.

"I wanted to tell you the miracle myself. I don't know how you did it, but this one is for the medical books. You had a possibility of seven eggs maximum from the last ultrasound—but we got fourteen!"

I burst into tears. I was so prepared for bad news that getting good news just pushed me over the edge.

"Seriously," he said, "Your body must have put in a triumphant effort in the last thirty-six hours, as none of us saw that coming. I don't think I have ever had an IVF round where we came that close to cancelling and then ended up here."

I actually didn't know how I felt. "Grateful" was one word that came to mind, but you get to a point where you are always waiting for the slap in the face.

"I recommend that we do ICSI on all fourteen," he said. "It's your best chance for fertilization."

I was about to agree and then something stopped me.

"No," I said. "I want some to be fertilized 'naturally.'" As much as putting sperm with an egg in a Petri dish is natural. Both Sam and Dr. T. started to argue with me.

"Why risk not fertilizing at this point?"

"I don't know," I said, "but I feel that if this baby is going to happen, it will happen without ICSI. ICSI feels like I'm forcing the issue."

Sam chimed in, "Julie, we've been forcing a baby for the last four years. Why the hell do you see this as being any different?" He was right, of course.

Dr. T. suddenly said, "You know, you need to do what is right for you. My recommendation is that we do all fourteen ICSI; but my recommendation last week was to cancel; we didn't and we got fourteen eggs."

"How about six natural and eight ICSI?" That was my compromise. "Sam, are you okay with that?"

"I've no clue," he said, "but so far what I think does not seem to matter, so do what you think."

I felt crappy; I knew Sam was angry, but I also felt strongly that "all ICSI" was not the right way to go.

"Okay, eight ICSI and six natural it is," I said and off went Dr. T.

"I hope you are right, " Sam said. I felt sick when he said that; I knew if this didn't work out that this decision would be revisited many times over, both spoken and unspoken.

"Me too," I said.

Sam could see that I was struggling with this and that the decision was now made, so he tried to focus on the fact that we had fourteen eggs this time. I reminded him that we still had a long way to go and that our fertilization rates were less than stellar.

"Yup," he said, "but it's better, Julie."

I really wanted to be enthusiastic, but couldn't be. I told Sam he had to take the call regarding the fertilization. I couldn't handle it.

They called twenty-four hours later. I saw the number, but didn't answer. I called Sam and said, "You have to call them. Every time they've called me, it's been bad news; we need to change our luck."

He called me back, "Guess what?" he said, "We have six fertilized eggs. Your theory is right, don't answer any more calls from the clinic; just direct them to me."

Apparently out of the fourteen eggs retrieved, eleven had been inseminated, and three were just duff, I guess. They did six naturally, but only two of those had fertilized. Of the five ICSI eggs, four had fertilized. I was beginning to regret my decision to split the eggs between "natural" and ICSI, versus going with all ICSI. Sam didn't have to say anything. I knew he was already regretting not fighting harder for ICSI.

However, two hurdles were down: number of eggs and the fertilization. The next deal breaker was the quality and grade. We were scheduled for the transfer on the Wednesday. This time, I wanted to know the grade of the eggs before I was on the table. Why a few minutes made any difference to me, I was not sure, but it did. I just felt really vulnerable hearing about the grade when I was lying down right before they inserted them. This time I refused to lie down and wanted to hear the grades sitting up.

The doctor—Dr. T. was not on duty—came in and I held my breath. I felt Sam stop breathing too.

"You won't believe this," he said, "but you have four relatively good eggs: a 10-cell, grade 2; an 8-cell, grade 2; an 8-cell, grade 4; and a 6-cell, grade 3. I only want to put three in, so I'm debating which will be the third, the 8-cell, grade 4 or the 6-cell, grade 3."

We decided on the 6-cell one.

He said, "I know your case and you should know that, of the three best eggs, we are transferring the two that fertilized naturally. So, whatever made you decide to split the fertilization, it was a good call. We're putting in two natural ones and one ICSI."

I think for the first time in a long time, I smiled. "Thank you," I said to no one in particular. To this day, I don't know what had made me make those decisions, but I smiled as I felt the universe was with me on this one.

The transfer was pretty uneventful. The only difference was this time the nurses hugged me and wished me all the best. The doctor didn't hug me, but he said, "This has been your best one. I know there are no guarantees, but good luck."

My next stop, straight after the transfer, was the acupuncturist. Sam waited for me while I had the treatment. The woman was great and after she finished she said, "Your womb feels warm," and again she gave me a hug. For a non-hugger like myself, this had been quite a huggy day and it made me feel like everyone was rooting for me. Also, I think I was so depleted that I couldn't resist it anymore.

I got in the car. I could see Sam had something on his mind (apart from the obvious!). "Thanks," he said.

"What for?" I asked.

"I don't know. You just kept going when I would have given up, and you didn't waver, even when everyone was telling you to do the opposite. Why was that?"

"I really don't know why, Sam. I think that what it came down to for me was ultimately the fact that I just truly knew I couldn't do it again; so I needed it to be over. Probably not what you wanted to hear, but I think that was what it was."

"Okay," he said. "No, not what I wanted to hear, but I'll buy it. Let's go get something to eat. I'm starving."

IVF #3

My Final IVF read like this:

Suppression drug: None—"IVF light"
Fertility drug: Puregon—10 days
Eggs: A whopping 14!
Fertilized: 6
Grades: Definitely better than terrible: 10-cell, grade 2; 8-cell, grade 2; 6-cell, grade 3
Result: Unknown at this point
Cost: $10,000 + psychic + fertility yoga + energy person + vision board + meditation CDs + more wine + therapy
Insanity scale: 9 out of 10. Finally lost it.
Relationship: 3 out of 10. Hanging on by a thread.

Make or Break

Two weeks after the eggs are transferred can be the most stressful time in the IVF process. Mainly, because there is absolutely nothing you can do at this point. You can't take any more drugs; you can't hope for a better egg to be inserted; it's done. Now, it's up to your body and, in my mind, the universe, to either create or not. This was our last IVF, so the stakes for me felt way higher; but I have to say at the same time there was a bit of relief, because if things did not work out, then I could move on with my life.

The reality of this meant that I would have to accept that children would not be a part of my life and also, after eleven years together, Sam and I would need to separate. I knew in my heart of hearts that I just couldn't handle another round of this. I felt I had been "stuck" for four years now and that was long enough. I think this is perhaps the hardest part of the IVF process— knowing when you personally have had enough.

Some couples and individuals can keep going. I heard about one woman who was on her twentieth time trying. I both admire that and also, in truth, struggle to understand it, because I am not built that way.

Two weeks after the transfer, I had to go in for the blood test. I was actually numb. Unlike IVF Numbers One and Two, the good news was that I had not started bleeding; but I also knew that didn't really mean anything, because my period could just have been late.

The nurses that help with IVF are a pretty incredible bunch. They know that the results of that blood test can cause a person extreme happiness or, in many cases, it can cause them to break. I remember one of the nurses very well; she was this beautiful, softly spoken, Asian nurse. She asked if this was my first, and I said, "No, it's my third and it's my last."

She said, "I guess it's now or never then."

"Yup." There really isn't any more they can say. She took the blood sample, which we both knew contained the answer to which way my life was going to go, and she simply said, "Good luck."

I thanked her for all her support and left. She labelled the test tube and sent it off to the lab. Walking away, I knew that it would be the last time I would visit that lab; a part of my life was over.

I went into work that morning. I should have mentioned that, after I had decided to quit my job in advertising, Christine, my friend who recommended the psychic, was in the process of creating a start-up called "DreamBank." It is a really neat idea; it takes away all the stress of gift giving, especially for group gifts and milestone birthdays. Customers just post online what they want as a gift, and friends and family can contribute as much or as little as they want toward the gift. For people like me who hate shopping and end up buying stuff nobody really wants, this is perfect. I really liked the idea so after quitting my ad agency job, I offered to help out at DreamBank. This was very much a part-time job to start with, but as we got closer to launching, it became more full-time. By the time I was waiting for the results of the final IVF, we were well into the peak of launching the start-up. No one in my workplace knew that I was going through IVF and I think that was the best thing for me.

The only person who did know was Christine, the CEO, and at this time she was in England finishing off her MBA. So it was me and the developer, Dave, trying to make sure we had everything covered. I like working with developers. They are an interesting bunch. They tend to have a real passion for what they are doing and they are often insanely bright and logical.

Going through a drug-induced hormonal state surrounded by guys who don't deal with emotion that well was a great relief to me. It kept me "restrained," as every time I felt I was on the edge of losing it, the thought of having a mini-breakdown in front of Dave conjured up such awkward images that they brought me back from the brink. I also remember avoiding going to the bathroom—I dreaded that I might see I had started my period.

Sam called at ten in the morning on the day we were meant to find out the test results. It went something like this:

Sam: "Well, have you called?"

Me: "No. I can't."

Sam: "Bloody hell, Julie. I've been sitting here thinking you knew and haven't told me, so I assumed it was bad news. Why haven't you called?"

Me: "I can't. I don't want to know. You call."

Sam: "Well, we need to find out either way. I don't want to call either, but one of us has to."

Me: "I know. You call. You have a better track record with telephone calls."

Sam: "Okay. I'll call you when I know."

Me: "I'm scared."

Sam: "Me too."

That hour before Sam called back was one of the most surreal hours in my life. I was torn between having a major meltdown in one of the adjoining offices, working slavishly on the launch of DreamBank, or just leaving the office altogether and never answering the phone again. There is something so strange in the time before you know that what you find out in the next while could change the trajectory of your life. It's like the universe wants you to remember what it is like to experience a moment of complete uncertainty and vulnerability.

The phone rang and I genuinely felt sick. This was the end of our journey to have kids, one way or another. In about ten seconds, I would have my answer. I went into another room, picked up the phone, and just started crying. I literally couldn't handle it anymore. I was expecting it to be another disappointment and knew that I didn't have the mental capacity to deal with it. I just sobbed.

Me: "It didn't work, did it?"

Sam: "It did."

Me: "What? Really? How do you know?"

Sam: "The HCG count is high."

Me: "What does that mean?"

Sam: "It means we're pregnant."

I actually can't remember what I said. I just cried. Cried because it had worked; cried because I was emotionally spent; cried because finally things had gone our way.

The next few days were pretty tense. In IVF you find out very early if you are pregnant. Each morning I would wake up thankful, but also fearing to start my period at any moment. When you actually get something that you have been struggling for, for what seems like an eternity, suddenly a whole new set of fears arise: what if you lose it? I think I was happy for about three days before I let all the new fears creep in. I think this may be a British trait—the glass is often half empty, very rarely half full.

I actually don't think I slept for the first two weeks after getting the results. It felt as though if I slept then something could happen that was out of my control, so it was best to stay vigilant at all times. Needless to say, I was knackered pretty quickly.

The only people we told were my sister, Maxine, and my friend Christine. I called Maxine as soon as I got the news.

She was delighted for me. It finally felt like at least one of us had some good news and I knew it was genuine. But she then let me know she was dealing with some fairly big stuff of her own. She was two years post-chemo and cancer-free, and her medical team had said that at the two-year mark they would discuss her options. I always thought you had to be five years free, but apparently not. Maxine was thirty-seven; she needed to make some tough decisions. Her options weren't great.

The oncologist told her that she could try for a baby, but there was a big downside. Because her cancer was so receptive to hormones, there was a chance that the cancer would return, as they would have to take her off the drugs she was on that were "keeping the hormones at bay." Plus, if it came back while she was pregnant, although she could be treated, it was risky. In their opinion, she could be risking her life if she decided to get pregnant. Her only real option, if she wanted a child without putting herself at risk, was surrogacy.

Maxine was angry. All along she had thought that once she was cancer-free, she would be able to have a baby. Beating cancer only to be told that after all you are still no closer to your dream is heartbreaking. Although an option, surrogacy was tough to consider. All that we knew then was that it could cost upwards of $70,000, was illegal in some states in the US, and there were no guarantees. Yes, it was an option, but it didn't feel like it at the time.

"What do you think?" she asked.

I didn't know what to say. "As a good friend, I don't want you to risk your life getting pregnant. I don't think that would be right for you or for the baby. Imagine giving birth to a child and then potentially either dying from cancer or having to go through chemo all over again in the first year of the baby's life. That would seriously suck, Maxine."

But I knew it was not my decision and she had to do what she thought was right. One of the worst things was they couldn't even give her exact statistics on the chance of the cancer returning, as the oncologist said there are not enough documented cases of this kind of cancer. I think in his mind the risk was too high.

"I guess, Maxine, what it comes down to is do you want to carry your baby, or do you just want a baby?"

"I really want a baby," she said, "but I'm mad about the fact that I don't have the option to carry it without risking my life."

Fair point. She had gone through enough and deserved a break.

"Well, have a think about it, Max. You know how I feel, but obviously it's up to you."

Over the next two weeks, I got off the fence. I called Maxine, as I was now adamant that carrying a child was not all it's cracked up to be. Here's why. About a week after we got the results, I was lying in bed and suddenly I started to feel strange. It was like someone was sitting on my chest and I couldn't breathe. I expected this when I became eight months pregnant, but not after fourteen days. I got up and went to the bathroom. I was very pale and looked like I was swelling up. I was having trouble breathing and felt very sick. Not having been pregnant before, I was not sure if this was normal or not, so I got back into bed. At 5:00 a.m. the next morning, I knew this wasn't normal. I had swelled up and looked like I was six months pregnant. I was dizzy and sweating. I was also frightened. I told Sam something was wrong and that I was going into the clinic. Sam had a meeting that morning so he couldn't come with me, but I could see he was concerned.

I managed to arrive at the clinic as it opened. They took me into a little room, weighed me, and measured my waist. I asked, "What is going on?"

They weren't one-hundred percent sure, but they thought it was something called ovarian hyperstimulation syndrome (OHSS). It is quite a rare condition, but I had a vague memory of reading about it as a risk of IVF. It occurs in about three to eight percent of the population. There is a range from mild to severe, but I won't bore you with the details. Essentially, I was already in the moderate to severe range. This means I was putting on approximately two pounds a day and my girth was expanding. The irony is that my sister also suffered from this condition. She was very severe and had to stay off work for about a month and just sit on the couch. This sounded perfect to me, but that was not going to happen. My doctor said, "This is actually a good sign: it means the pregnancy has likely taken hold. But you need to weigh yourself and measure your girth every morning and call in with the measurements, so we know if we need to hospitalize you. If possible, please rest up at home."

I did stay at home for a few days, but we were launching a company and I knew there were a lot of things on my plate that had to get done, so I called the doctor and asked if I could go back to work. My girth measurements had levelled off and my blood pressure was normal so he gave me the okay, but said to call him if anything changed.

Now, here's the dilemma. The last time Dave the developer had seen me, I was a reasonably normal, middle of the range, thirty-nine-year-old. Now, I looked like I was a six-months pregnant thirty-nine-year-old. So I needed to come up with an explanation and a "miraculous" six-month-old baby in my belly was not going to cut it.

I said that I had a kidney infection and was bloated with fluid. I still remember the look on his face when I came in. "Whoa!" were the first words out of his mouth. "I thought you were kidding when you said you looked six-months pregnant. You underestimated. You look like you're about to give birth."

Guys! I just love them, don't you? Then it was back to launching DreamBank as per normal. Dave kept looking over at me and shaking his head.

I said, "Do you want to touch it?"

That shut him up.

I called Maxine and said, "Maxine, this hasn't really been my week. I couldn't breathe; spent nearly a day in the clinic; feel completely nauseous; have to weigh and measure myself every day; and pretend I have a kidney infection so no one will question why I look like the side of a house. You know how you asked me earlier what I thought, well, here's what I think: carrying the baby is not the point; it is ending up with one. Being pregnant is just a means to an end and so far my experience has not been great. I know surrogacy is a very tough option and perhaps impossible, but I am not prepared to lose you as a friend. So I hope you decide not to carry your own child. Plus, Maxine, let's be honest; you're one of my vainest friends and having you call me complaining every week about how your body is changing is not something I would look forward to."

I don't think I gave her the chance to respond. She called back later. "Okay," she said, "if Tom agrees, we will think about surrogacy." I think she had already come to this conclusion herself, but my rant may have helped push her along.

"Good," I said. "If you would like me to call to tell him about

the downside of pregnancy to help support your decision, I will."
I didn't have to.

She came to see me when I was about five-months pregnant, saw the state of me, and, drinking a glass of wine said, "You know, Ju, you don't look that good."

Really, Maxine? Really?

Maxine was a champion, though. I felt it was unfair that I was having to go through my struggles, but it didn't compare to what Maxine was dealing with. It's a cliché, but there is always someone worse off than yourself. I'm sure Maxine, like many of us, had some very dark moments when she probably hit rock bottom. I had an occasional glimpse into this when I think she just needed to vent; but she refused to be a victim in all of this and she never gave up. I'm not sure I would have had the strength she found. At no point that I can remember did she ever say, "I'm done." She often said, "I need a break," but she was going to have a baby, come hell or high water. Her journey in some ways was just starting and she was a long way from the finish line.

Slowly, my OHSS condition of looking six-months pregnant when I wasn't got under control; but for the first few weeks of the pregnancy, I felt very fragile. I knew all the statistics about how anything can happen and I was more vulnerable to miscarriage in the time before twelve weeks, just like any "normal" pregnancy. I was designated the status of "geriatric mother." I thought that was a joke, but apparently, no. Over the age of thirty-five in Canada, first-time pregnant women are classified as "geriatric." I found out that, in England, they stopped using this term in the Eighties and now use the term "elderly *primagravida.*" Is putting part of it in Latin really that much better?

Either way, the medical world saw me as old and probably, from a fertility perspective, I was, but I really didn't need to see it on my medical sheet. I think they may need to change that term in the near future, because women are having babies at even older ages, so they are going to have to change the criteria or come up with something a little more palatable.

Who the hell thinks up these labels, anyway? I found out. When I was ranting about the above to a very funny nurse I met on one appointment, she said, "You haven't heard the half of it. There are a few terms like that around in the medical profession. If you miscarry many times you are called a 'habitual aborter' and if your cervix is too short it is called an 'incompetent cervix!'"

She then added very dryly, "Can't you tell it was men who invented these terms?"

I did laugh because she was right. I'm sure if females had developed those terms they would not be the same. We would likely have ended up with something like "cervix that needs support," and as for "geriatric," how about "mothers who believe they are much younger than they really are and who didn't want to give up drinking wine until the last possible moment." I'm half-joking here, but basically, I think it's time to change these labels.

Nausea hit me pretty hard right from the get-go. I was definitely not prepared for that. Feeling sick all the time, every day, was hard. Working, feeling sick, and still coping with OHSS was definitely a struggle for me. But feeling sick was a good sign, the doctors said, so I sucked it up (well, not literally) and got on with it.

I was moaning to Maxine about things one particularly bad day and in true Maxine fashion she said, "Julie, remember chemo."

"Okay, you win yet again on the misery front," I replied.

My date was scheduled for the six-week scan. When the day arrived, I put on my lucky pink t-shirt. This was the t-shirt that I had worn for a lot of the last IVF, and because it looked like it had worked, I decided to wear it for all the hospital appointments. I'm sure the staff must have thought that was the only t-shirt I had. Even Sam said at one point, "Ju, all I've seen you in for the last six weeks is that t-shirt. Don't you have anything else?"

I had to explain that this was my LUCKY t-shirt, with a big emphasis on the word "lucky." If I changed my t-shirt then I might put on the UNLUCKY t-shirt by mistake and we just don't want to risk that, do we? Sam was smart. He just kept quiet.

I was throwing up in the car park, just before we went in for the scan. I felt terrible. If nausea was a sign that the baby was "sticking," this one was super-glued to the wall. Waiting for the scan, I really wanted to enjoy the moment. We were finally pregnant, had made it to six weeks, and so far so good; but I was anxious. Sam was calm yet I could feel some of his excitement, so I focused on that. I had to drink quite a bit of water and the wait time was quite long. I noticed this is a theme in the medical world when it comes to some ultrasounds. They ask you to drink a lot then make you wait beyond the point of pain, and then, as happened with me, my super-large bladder was so full that it obscured the screen and we couldn't see the uterus!

I had to go and "pee just a little," as if it's possible to pee a little when you're desperate to go with a bladder that is full to the brim. It was like trying to stop the great flood. My Kegel exercises had obviously failed miserably.

When I got back, I explained to the ultrasound nurse that, unfortunately, my bladder was probably quite empty now. He didn't seem too fussed. He was very quiet and didn't say anything at all while scanning me.

There is one thing I distinctly remember, but to this day, have still not gotten to the bottom of it. He asked me something like, "Do you have a split cervix?"

Personally, I had never heard of this, so I couldn't really answer. I said, "I have no clue. What is it?"

He said that the cervix can split into two and sometimes the uterus splits as well, so a woman could have a two-chambered uterus. This all sounded a bit freakish to me. He thought there might be something a little odd about my cervix, but it was not clear; and if no one else had picked up on it, after having about a million ultrasounds with IVF, then we thought it was nothing to worry about.

Amazingly, I had to pee again, as obviously my humungous bladder was not in fact empty. I excused myself quickly after he had finished, as I couldn't hold on any longer. I came back in and Sam looked shocked. I panicked and asked, "What's wrong?"

He just held up three fingers and said, "There are three."

I sat down on the bed and said, "Three what?"

"Three sacs."

I wasn't comprehending "sacs," so I said, "You mean three babies?"

He nodded. I started crying. I was completely overwhelmed. All this time, after everything we had tried, just having one child seemed like a monumental struggle, and now I was hearing there were three. We had never even contemplated at this point having more than one child. The technician could see that this was a big shock. His bedside manner was not the best; but he showed us the sacs and the heartbeats. He said, "You have two very strong heart beats and one much weaker heartbeat, which may not make it."

This was a lot to take in. Three babies, not one, and one which looked as though it might not make it. We were both in shock when we left and we sat in the car. I was still crying and Sam was very quiet. He said, "This should be the happiest moment of our lives and it feels overwhelming. I'm happy, but how the hell are we going to cope with three children, no family support, and living in an apartment?"

There were many times during my pregnancy when I wanted a big glass of wine and this was one of them.

At least it explained the severe morning sickness.

Next was to have another scan at eight weeks to see how things were progressing. The news of multiples is how I obtained my new title of "high-risk geriatric mother." Being forty at birth with potential triplets catapults you into a whole different level. Firstly, I was assigned an obstetrician. I actually had no idea what they did. Basically, they specialize in childbirth. Secondly, the other benefit of this, as there has to be one, is that if you are old and a carrier of multiple sacs, you often get pushed to the front of the queue.

The downside is that this news comes with a whole load of possible complications. Once the news was settling in, I started to try and figure out what this would mean in terms of the pregnancy. Between the family doctor, the obstetrician, and Google, I submerged myself in a world of frightening statistics. There are of course variations, but on the whole, here's how it reads (all from sources on Google):

- Pregnancy-induced hypertension (PIH) is high blood pressure during pregnancy. As many as 37% of twin pregnancies involve PIH, which is three to four times the rate in singleton pregnancies (*www.pregnancy.about.com/od/hypertensionpre/a/pihinpg.htm*).
- Pre-eclampsia is a condition that includes both high blood pressure and protein in the urine. It is twice as likely to occur in mothers of multiples (*www.pregnancy.about.com/od/pqr/g/preeclampsia.htm*).
- Mothers of multiples are more likely to experience postpartum depression (*www.depression.about.com/cs/babyblue/a/postpartumdep.htm*).
- Preterm birth is much more likely with multiples—the average gestational length for singletons is thirty-nine weeks; for twins thirty-five weeks; and for triplets thirty-one weeks. This can be an issue, as premature births often come with complications because some organs, like the lungs, are often not fully developed.

The list went on and on. It was brutal and scary. There is also a whole different level of complications if the twins share a placenta or are in the same sac and so on. As far as we knew, all ours had separate sacs and placentas so this was helpful, but still the statistics were intimidating.

Even for me—someone who likes to know all the facts—this was overwhelming. I read all about it. Then, once I felt I knew the risks, I shut down my computer, decided we would deal with it as best we could, and also decided that fate would probably have to take over. The alternative was that I would become a neurotic basket case. And that would not do me, the babies, nor my relationship with Sam any good at all.

The eight-week scan came along. We had an appointment with the fertility clinic after this one, as essentially this would be where we shook hands, they would say, "Our job is done," and we would part. I was much calmer for the eight-week scan as I was slowly accepting the fact that life really was going to change dramatically, so we might as well get used to it. Plus, I wanted to see how my three monkeys were doing.

Well, two monkeys were doing well, but the third monkey hadn't made it. There was no longer a heartbeat. We had learned there was a high risk of this, but it was still hard to hear.

I asked what would happen to the third monkey. Would I miscarry it? And would that mean I might risk the other two? This is where I learned something new. The nurse explained that, no, at the stage of development that the third fetus was, my body would reabsorb it.

To me, that was incredible! The body is so smart! It also made me feel a little better, as I thought it would still be a part of me and his/her other two monkeys. Sometimes, I have to trust that my body knows what is best for me. This was reinforced when we went for our final appointment with Dr. T. at the fertility clinic.

He first congratulated us and then he said, "These guys are the miracle babies. I hope you don't mind my saying so, but I never thought, based on the way the last IVF went, that we would end up with this result. I mean, we were going to cancel. I'm going to use your story—with your permission—just so people know that sometimes what happens doesn't make sense, and sheer hope and faith seem to be the only explanation."

He then added, "I'm actually relieved the third monkey didn't make it." Well, he didn't call it a monkey—I can't imagine what that would have done to his medical reputation if he had. "If you continued to carry three, pending on a few things, we most likely would have suggested a selective reduction where we remove one embryo, just because the risk of triplets at your age might have compromised both your health and the health of the other two."

There are times in my life when I have been eternally grateful and this was one of them. I understand the logic of "selective reduction" and also the reasons why people may choose to do it, but, thank God, I didn't have to make that choice. Deciding to eliminate a life to save potentially three others makes sense, but having to choose to do it raises an emotional, ethical, "no-right answer," and, in my mind, "no-win" decision.

We thanked Dr. T. He had undoubtedly been the right choice for us. He had listened; he had been honest, sincere, and had a great sense of humour. He had supported us (or me!) in every request, regardless of how bizarre or irrelevant he thought it was, and in the end he had got us pregnant. I hugged him. He wished us luck. He said we would need it with twins....

So we were now officially having twins. We were eight-weeks pregnant and we thought it was time to tell our closest family. My Mum and sister Jane with her IVF-miracle-son Henry were out for a holiday in Vancouver. Jane knew already, but she had not told our Mum, as she wanted it to be a surprise.

A little bit about our Mum. She is an amazing human being who has such a caring capacity, and although she has rheumatoid arthritis and a lung condition, not unlike cystic fibrosis (but not life-threatening), she still manages to care for many others. At this point in my journey, she was looking after Ken across the road, who has a mental illness; her own Mum of ninety-four; a ninety-year-old neighbour; my sister's little boy, during the day; the two dogs of a close family member; and pretty much anyone else who needs it. It always conjures up an amusing image for me. My Mum, who sometimes struggles to walk, saying she is off to do the vacuuming for the neighbour, as the neighbour is not finding things as easy as they used to be.

Her life has not been easy. She lost my Dad about a month into his retirement. They were one of the happiest couples I knew and his death was like a cannon ball smashing through her life. It nearly broke her. I remember how she seemed to just withdraw from life. She really did lose a part of herself when Dad died. They were so looking forward to their retirement together. I'm still angry about my Dad's death for a number of reasons, but mainly because my Mum needed him. But my Mum was and is a survivor and despite her grief, she was still getting up every day. I am not sure how she did it, but she did. And she still does.

My Mum had also given up on me and Jane ever having children. She also officially gave up on me ever getting married. One day she announced that she had thrown out everything she had collected for me relating to the "bottom drawer" (i.e. savings for a wedding), and said, "Here's a cheque. Use it for what you want."

I hadn't even known she had saved a "bottom drawer" for me. At least she's practical; I like that. Thank goodness Jane finally got married at thirty-seven and had produced a grandchild at forty-two! Dad died before Jane got married, so he never met her husband, Henry, or Sam, and he wouldn't meet my twins either. I think that's why I'm still a bit angry.

Having Mum, Jane and Henry here was great, except I had to pretend I wasn't feeling like throwing up every five minutes. It was probably the worst period of nausea I'd ever had. I told Mum I just had a stomach bug, and she totally believed me. Mind you, she did point out one day that I spent a lot of time in sweat pants and my pink t-shirt. Ah, little did she know that it was my LUCKY pink t-shirt and that until I got to three months at least, it was staying very much close to my side.

Mum had her seventieth birthday while she was visiting. My brilliant birthday plan was to send Mum skydiving off Grouse Mountain and then tell her we were having twins. If that wasn't a birthday to remember, then I didn't know what would be. Sam kindly pointed out that she was seventy and had rheumatoid arthritis, so maybe we should just go out for dinner instead. Fair point, but once I have an idea, I tend to see it through, good or bad.

Much to our amazement, once she was over the shock that she was going to be launched off a mountain, Mum was completely into it. She loved it.

I then gave her her birthday card. It said, "I know that it has been a long time coming, but I thought I'd let you know you are now going to have three grandchildren."

Mum was stunned, "Are you serious?" she asked.

"Yup," I said.

In typical Mum fashion, she said to Jane and me, "Really you two. Couldn't you have done this earlier? I'm seventy-years-old and now you decide to have three children in the space of eighteen months. Good God, could you have left it any later? I won't have any energy to look after them."

Cheers, Mum! It actually wasn't for lack of trying. Funnily enough, it is amazing how much energy a seventy-year-old can find.

Sam's parents were equally thrilled. They had very generously offered to help cover some of the costs of this final IVF and we were very grateful. I think they secretly thought that I didn't want kids and that they were also never going to be grandparents. I can't blame them; we never really told anyone the full details of what we were going through, so people just came to their own conclusions. I would have done the same. Sam is an only child. He was under a lot of pressure. He was the last in his line of Dexters, so the future of the family name was resting on his shoulders. I mean, could you imagine a world of no more Dexters? It was totally unthinkable! I think Sam shielded me from a lot of the "continuation of the line" and "we'll lose our spot on ancestry.com" conversations. For that, I am appreciative.

Now, the plan was to sit tight and keep our fingers crossed. The next big hurdle was the NT scan. "NT" stands for nuchal translucency scan. This is a scan of the fluid behind the babies' necks. It can indicate a chromosomal abnormality. For me, this test was a real stress point. I knew, as I was older, that my chances of having a child with an abnormality increased and I also knew logically that because I was carrying two, the chances increased again.

When I sit and think about this test, I am amazed how incredibly smart some individuals are. I mean, who managed to connect the fact that the depth of fluid in the neural tube was an indicator of potential chromosomal issues? Mind you, I am still astounded by Sir Alexander Bell who spent a large part of his life figuring out the telephone. How do those thoughts come into people's heads? Was he posting a letter and thought, "Jeez, there must be a faster way," and then, "I know, let's try and send sound down a wire." Incredible. Don't get me started on the internet. Tim Berners-Lee, the inventor of the World Wide Web is the epitome of genius, in my mind. For the record, the inventor of the NT scan is a world-leading research clinic run by Professor Nicolaides of the Fetal Medical Centre in London.

They told me the test results right away. The results for both babies looked okay. They stressed that it was approximately seventy-five to eight-five percent accurate, so we needed to decide if we were to have an amniocentesis (where they inject a needle into the amniotic fluid to test if there are any major chromosomal abnormalities), because that would be closer to ninety-nine percent accurate.

I actually had no problem with the idea of having an amnio test. Most pregnant couples I knew had had the test and everything went fine. There are some risks, but they are minimal in terms of chances of miscarrying. The statistics I read were less than one percent.

At this point, both Sam and I were open to the amnio, but before we had to make that decision, we had to undergo genetic counselling. I asked the clinic why we had to do this. They said that they offer this because there is potentially an increased risk of abnormalities in babies born via the ICSI method, some minor, some major. I read a lot about this. The information I found on my infertility buddy, Google, seemed to match what they said. I believe the jury is still out on the medical repercussions of ICSI, but I'll let the medical community debate that one.

Genetic counselling was interesting. First, she went through our own history. My side of the family is a bit of a disaster: my Dad was one of five. My Dad's Dad had died of a heart attack at the age of forty-four. My Dad had his first heart attack at a bar at age forty-four. He actually died; but was incredibly lucky that a nurse was in the bar at the time, and brought him back to life. The doctors had been concerned that because of this, my Dad would have had brain damage. I remember being eleven and thinking, "Oh no, I don't want a brain-damaged Dad." Totally selfish, I know, and I loved my Dad, but I know, for me as an eleven-year-old, this was a real concern. He had some memory issues for a while, but his memory came back slowly. His life changed though and the next few years were particularly tough. Dad couldn't work, we had little money, and my Mum was trying to hold it all together.

There was more—my Dad's brother also died from a heart attack before the age of sixty-five. His two sisters and his Mum died of cancer between the ages of sixty-nine and seventy-one. My Mum's side is a little more resilient. I remember saying to the counsellor, "It's not the best pedigree. Let's hope the kids get Sam's genes. Ha, ha, ha."

I thought I was being quite funny, but she said seriously, "Yes, you're right, that's not a pretty picture. You need to keep an eye on your health, too. You're having twins."

Great, now I was paranoid that I was going to keel over in my early forties. Sam's side of course was much more impressive. A couple of strokes and an incidence of cancer; nothing too much to blight the Dexter pedigree. Typical.

Part of the discussion during the genetic counselling was to help us determine whether we should go ahead with the amniocentesis. Here is the rub in my opinion with the amnio. You first need to decide what you would do with the results. If the results were problematic, would we take action so we could prepare for any issues that might arise? If we were doing it just to find out and not sure what we would do with the results, then it is recommended that you figure that out first!

We didn't know what we would do with the results. And to make matters worse, with twins (no surprises here!), if you do decide to undergo an amnio, the chances of miscarriage double as there are two.

And here is the bit that really got me. If we were to decide that we would abort the fetus if there were issues, then with twins—where one is okay and one is not—there is a very real possibility that we might lose the wrong baby because they move around so much that it's hard to be one-hundred percent sure. Apparently, this actually happened where a mother of twins decided to abort the one with poor amnio results, but the medical team actually aborted the healthy child.

Sam and I went home. Here is another moment when I wanted a large glass of wine! Sometimes during my pregnancy I wish I lived in Europe, because although they don't encourage drinking during pregnancy, they are a tad more lenient if you do want to treat yourself, every now and again.

This decision raised a lot of questions. To risk losing both babies for the sake of this test felt like too big of a risk to take; but it was also a bit daunting to consider having twins with potentially one or both with challenges, no family support, and both of us having to work to cover our bills.

I have a cousin with Down's Syndrome who is an awesome individual and has been the light of my aunty and uncle's lives, but my aunty was always a stay-at-home Mum so she could devote her energies to him and her other four children. We didn't know if we could make it work in our situation. There was also the other end of the argument, where it would be better to know what we were dealing with so we could be prepared.

We had many sleepless nights over this. The genetic counsellor was amazing. She was at a conference in Halifax, but she returned my calls and gave me as much information as possible. In the end, I said, "If you were me, with everything you have seen and know, what would you do?"

Her answer was, "Well, based on what you have been through to get here, the results of the NT scan and the potential risk of miscarrying, I would likely not do the amnio. But the real question is, if something were to go wrong and you lost them, would you be able to forgive yourself? Also," she said, "there is also a nineteen-week scan when, although this is a tough route, if there are any issues, there is still the chance you can selectively reduce your pregnancy. At nineteen weeks, there is a much lower chance that you would lose both babies, as they are better established."

See? I told you she was good. For probably only the second time in my life, I relinquished this to the universe. Bottom line, Sam and I could not face it if we miscarried the twins as a result of this decision, so we just trusted that we would be able to deal with whatever the outcome would be. However, as the date for when we needed to do the amnio approached and passed, we both inwardly went over the decision many times in our heads again.

I was now starting to relax. I was fourteen-weeks pregnant and the concept that we might actually end up with these two babies was seeding in my mind. I can't say I was enjoying the pregnancy. For about seven weeks I had endured what I would call the "mother of all migraines." This headache was unlike any headache I had ever experienced. I woke up with it. I went to bed with it. It kept me awake most nights. I slowly felt like I was going crazy. The doctors couldn't figure out what it was. I couldn't take anything for it and it was a constant distraction. My blood pressure was fine, so it was a real mystery. This went on for eight weeks total and then one morning, I woke up and, voila, I had my life back.

I felt sorry for Sam during this period. Everyone says that you should keep having regular sex throughout your pregnancy … yeah right! Morning sickness throughout the day, OHS syndrome, a permanent headache for eight weeks, tender boobs, nosebleeds, and hormonal overload! I don't think he really minded not having sex with me, because I didn't have the energy to shave my legs or anything, which probably meant I wasn't the most attractive proposition.

I continued having my regular checkups at the obstetrician's. Every two weeks, I had to go and have my cervix checked. Remember the "incompetent cervix"? Well, it's a big deal during pregnancy with twins. The length of my cervix was closely watched as—I realized—it is the plug that keeps everything in. I also had an ultrasound to check heartbeats. I have to say even though I'd had so many ultrasounds, I still couldn't recognize what they were pointing to on the screen. They would say, "Can you see that is the arm?" or foot, or whatever, and I would duly say "Umm, I think so." But I can honestly say that, until near the end, I couldn't recognize anything. Especially with two, there is little room to get a clear picture, but I trusted that these people had seen enough to identify the relevant body parts.

The Home Stretch

We still hadn't told anyone outside close family and a couple of friends about the pregnancy. I just didn't want to tempt fate. This actually came back to bite me. At about sixteen weeks, we decided to venture more than four blocks from our house. We had stuck to four blocks just in case there was an emergency. Six blocks would probably have been okay, too, but we were conservative.

We booked a weekend away with two of our friends, Rob and Mary. We headed off for a relaxing weekend to Sechelt on the Sunshine Coast. This was about a forty-five-minute car journey and a forty-minute ferry ride away. My biggest stress was about how I would cover up the fact that I was not drinking, as these were my food-and-wine buddies. Ah ha, the good old bladder infection. It's a good one. Guys are too uncomfortable to ask questions and girls screw up their faces and cross their legs in sympathy, as they have more-than-likely experienced one in their lifetimes.

We arrived on a Friday and had booked dinner for that evening. The memories of this night are tattooed on my grey matter forever. I say tattooed versus etched or imprinted, as neither of those reflect the pain and anxiety that was to come. We were just checking into the restaurant when I felt something warm trickle down my leg. I froze. Then I rushed to the washroom, closed my eyes, and pulled down my trousers. I didn't want to open my eyes as I was scared about what I might see. But I had to. There was bright red blood everywhere. I nearly collapsed. This could not be happening. Not after all we had been through. No! No! Nooooo!

I managed to stuff my knickers full of toilet paper to soak it up and went outside. Sam was waiting for me, as the others were at the table, and he could sense that something was wrong. "I'm bleeding," I told him.

"Shit," was all he said. We then had to tell Rob and Mary that: a) we were pregnant; b) we were pregnant with twins; and c) I was bleeding quite heavily and needed to go to the hospital.

Rob and Mary were both shocked and supportive. They came to the hospital while I waited to be admitted. The whole process took a long time. They fell asleep in the car while waiting. Eventually, Sam went outside and said it looked like it was going to be a long night, so they should try and get a taxi home, and we would see them as soon as we could.

They wheeled me into the emergency room. I explained that I was pregnant and we had done IVF. The nurse was pretty straightforward. "You are bleeding quite a lot and the blood is fresh, so there is a high chance that you are miscarrying."

I felt completely hollow. I looked at Sam and I could see he was devastated. After all we had been through, it was going to end in a hospital room in Sechelt.

I said, "How can you tell for sure?" There was a very strong part of me that refused to believe this was happening.

She said that the only real way to tell was to detect the babies' heartbeats. For the next five minutes she tried to detect the heartbeats with a hand device she kept running over my stomach. She detected a heartbeat, but she didn't know if it belonged to me or one of the babies.

"Can we do an ultrasound?" I asked, as I knew that would tell us for sure.

She said, "No, we only have ultrasound technicians available at certain times." It was a small hospital and there was no one on shift. I tried to be polite, but I wanted to scream the house down.

I said, "I don't bloody care, call him or her, and get them down here. I can't go through the night not knowing. Sam will go personally to pick them up, but please do something."

She said she couldn't and nature would just have to play out how it was going to be.

I didn't want bloody nature to "play it out." Nature, to date, had not been my best buddy and I wanted to know if I was going to lose my babies. Give me the friggin' ultrasound machine and I'll find the heartbeats. Needless to say, that approach did not get me very far.

I was still bleeding when I left the hospital (still without ultrasound). The blood seemed to have slowed by the time we reached the accommodation where we had to fill Rob and Mary in on all the details. They didn't really know what to say, as you would expect. I could barely talk, so I went to bed, pulled the covers over myself, and prayed as hard as I had ever prayed in my life. We decided we had to get back to Vancouver as soon as possible, so we left at the crack of dawn and got the first ferry back. We didn't say much to each other on the journey home. We knew that once again both the pregnancy and our future were in the balance. The one thing I do remember Sam saying was, "We're not going to lose these babies." I can't say I felt as positive as him, but I was grateful for his resolve.

We arrived at the hospital and were admitted to emergency. It was a slow day and the doctor on duty came to see me fairly quickly. He heard the background and then asked to take a look. I nearly jumped off the bed when he inserted his finger inside me. He pulled it out and said, "Yes, there is a lot of pooled blood and, without an ultrasound, it looks like it could be the start of a miscarriage. But the good news is that a lot of the blood is old, and there is very little fresh blood, which is an encouraging sign." He then proceeded to tell me the straight goods, "You have a one-in-five chance of miscarrying at your age and at this trimester with a multiple pregnancy." I like facts, but I needed to know if we still had one or two babies.

This doctor was incredible. He knew what we had been through and wanted to get us answers as soon as possible. There was no one in ultrasound, so he called a colleague, explained the situation, and asked if she could quickly do an ultrasound and help us out. She agreed. The doctor walked me down to the ultrasound.

I was holding Sam's hand so tightly. He looked pale, but I could still see his resolve. I got on the table and my whole body started shaking. It was probably the effects of no sleep, high anxiety, and just plain fear. They started the ultrasound. I held my breath. I remember the nurse saying after about thirty seconds, "We've got one!" referring to a heartbeat. The tears starting coming and it seemed like ages before she said, "Here's the other!"

I lost it and started crying and shaking at the same time. Both our little miracles were still alive. Even the doctor and nurse were excited for us. In the end they thought it had been a burst capillary or vein. I hung onto Sam all the way out, tears still pouring down my cheeks. We got home, phoned Rob and Mary to tell them the good news, went to bed, and passed out.

And—just for those of you who are not superstitious—guess what I was wearing when they found the two heartbeats? Yup, my LUCKY pink t-shirt. Even Sam didn't question it any more, and I wore it for every appointment thereafter.

The rest of my pregnancy was relatively smooth compared to the first half, except for the fact that I got pretty big. So big in fact that at one point apparently one of my ribs "unhinged," which itself put me in complete agony for about four weeks due to the fact that the babies were positioned really high in my body. I have small hips, so I guess they decided to head north, in search of roomier pastures. It's funny: many women get what they call *linea nigra*, which is a brown line running from the belly button down to the pubic area; it's caused by hormones. I had a *reversa linea nigra*: mine went north instead of south! Luckily for me, it disappeared later.

All I can remember toward the end of my pregnancy was there were lots of appointments. With twins it seems some crazy things can happen near the time of birth and it is not uncommon for there to be some serious complications.

A close friend of mine, Andrea, was unfortunate to have suffered one such serious complication. Andrea had also been pregnant with twins. They shared the same placenta and sac, and at thirty-six weeks, she went for an ultrasound and sadly learned that one of the babies had died. This is so heartbreaking, as you have to give birth to both, care for the surviving one, but also grieve for the lost twin. An impossible situation. Getting through each day must have been a battle.

I went to the funeral even though I was torn, because I wanted to show my support for her and her husband, but I didn't want to make her uncomfortable in any way. I had never been to a child's funeral. I can unequivocally say that it was one of the saddest things I have ever experienced. You can't help but question, "Why?" But there are no answers, or none that make any sense.

At nineteen weeks, we went for an ultrasound. This was the ultrasound that showed if there were any abnormalities as a second check to the NT scan. I was a little nervous, but because we had made our decision, we were going to live with whatever happened. We had to see the genetic counsellor straight after. The results looked encouraging, but until we gave birth, we would not know for sure. I also asked whether we could know the sex. She said she couldn't tell me, as in this province they want to avoid religious factors that can lead to decisions to abort based on sex. I said that was not the case with us, but didn't want to compromise her integrity. So in a stroke of genius, I said, "I know you can't tell us, but can you answer a question?"

"Yes," she said.

"Okay, are they both the same?"

She laughed and said, "No; good question."

So we knew we were having a boy and a girl.

As I said before, Sam is the last in the line of the Dexters, so although his parents didn't really care at this point—they were just glad to know they would soon be grandparents—I knew they were hoping deep down to continue their male line with a grandson.

We called them and I said, "Guess what! We're having twin girls!" There was a split second of silence on the phone while I think they composed themselves. Then Sam's Mum said, "Oh ...

that's great, really great. We've never had girls, have we, Harry?" I couldn't help but smile. They were genuinely pleased, but couldn't quite hide a tiny bit of disappointment. I quickly put them out of their misery. "Just kidding. It's one of each; the Dexter line lives to see another day." Their second reaction was a little different.

Virtually every three to five days toward the end, I was at the OB/GYN measuring my cervix or at the hospital monitoring heartbeats. My cervix was tested and measured more times than I care to remember. It was impressive though. There was no "shortening"; an "Olympian cervix," they called it. Nothing was going to get through this puppy.

The obstetrician advised me to go no longer than thirty-eight-and-a-half weeks due to potential complications. I said, "sure," because at this point I was uncomfortable enough and wanted to know that by thirty-eight-and-a-half weeks I would be done. She asked if I wanted a natural birth.

"Nothing about this pregnancy has been natural. Whatever is the safest way to get these out works for me. If I give birth naturally before thirty-eight weeks, no problem. If not, let's book a C-section."

The heartbeat monitoring was stressful. Knowing what my friend Andrea had been through, I was always tense at these appointments. There was always one beat that was hard to find. At one point, I had four people trying to find it. This is when I just had to lie there and keep calm. I remember thinking that there is a joke in here somewhere. "How many hospital staff does it take to find a heartbeat?" But really, I just kept telling myself it was all going to be all right.

I know some women cherish natural childbirth. But I have to say for me, if it had happened, great! But actually getting my head around giving birth to two babies was a bit freaky. Especially as, having Googled it to death, I could see there were often more complications in twin births, of course! I decided that if they didn't come before thirty-eight-and-a-half weeks, it was a sign that they wanted to come out by C-section.

Not long after the nineteen-week ultrasound, I got a call from Kari. I was number five in my core group of seven friends to get pregnant. Kari and Maxine were the last ones standing. I had told Kari, as soon as I could, that I was pregnant, as I really didn't want her hearing it from anyone else. I knew how tough it was hearing other people's positive news when you were on the edge of despair. She took it well and there were a few tears from both sides, because I knew she was so glad for me, but that doesn't stop the stab of pain you feel when you hear that yet another person is going to have a baby.

I asked her how the adoption process was going. "Slow," she said, but the good news was that Vietnam had opened up again, and that was their chosen country. So they were pursuing it full throttle in case it closed down again. The paperwork sounded horrendous and the emotional energy it took to go through the process sounded as bad as the IVF process.

So when she called to see if we could meet one day, I thought it was for her to give me an update on where they were at. I entered the coffee shop and saw her sitting there. She looked stressed, so I hoped it wasn't bad news for her.

"Hey," I said, "What's up?"

"Wow," she replied. "You are huge."

I had always liked her honesty. It was refreshing. Brutal, but refreshing! She said they had heard from the adoption agency and there were a pair of Vietnamese twins who had suddenly come up for adoption. Kari was in a total dilemma. She was forty-four at the time and didn't know if she could cope with twins. To remind you, Kari's husband is very successful and she had had a successful career as a designer herself. Then as her husband's job responsibilities had increased, her role had switched in the interim to being a supportive wife and partner. Her life was not perfect by any means, but she appreciated the freedom her lifestyle was able to afford her and self-admittedly had a low threshold for stress.

"Could I cope?" she asked.

"Don't ask me! I have no idea what it's going to be like. Hellish is my best guess, but Kari, this may be your only chance to adopt, so why not take it? You have always wanted two children and let's face it, you are not getting any younger. Your choice is to have two kids at forty-four, or one at forty-four, and then potentially another at forty-seven! Seriously, would you really want to adopt another at forty-seven, after having been through this process once? What does your husband think?"

"He wants us to go for it for all the same reasons, but he won't be the one looking after them and I'm scared that it will be too much."

"You will cope and if you can't, you can get help. Kari, I think you should do it. You've waited over ten years for a child. You don't want to do IVF and I don't want to mention age again, but you are forty-four!! There is not going to be a better chance. You have to take it. It probably is going to be a nightmare, but fortunately we both like wine, so I'm sure we'll be able to get through it."

"You're right," she said. I couldn't help but laugh. Here we were, the two oldest, the ones who had been trying for the longest, probably in truth the least maternal at the outset, and we were now both potentially having twins. The irony was not lost on us.

That night she called. "We're doing it," she said.

"Great! Keep me posted and best of luck."

I then got an email with pictures of the twins. They were beautiful. I had every bone crossed in my body that this would work out for her. It did. Three months after saying yes to the twins and after so many years of wanting a child, Kari and her husband arrived home from Vietnam, exhausted and overwhelmed, but with two of the most precious children for whom they had waited a lifetime. Only Maxine was left, but by all accounts, it looked like it might not happen for her.

In the meantime, we had to start getting ready. Most people I think who are not in the "unfertile" category start planning for the baby's arrival well in advance. Not so, I think, with the unfertiles. Until the babies get here, we don't like to take anything for granted. This, however, has its downsides. We didn't really start getting ready till week thirty-five. Not so smart. Trying to run around, research, paint, and write countless lists when you are grumpy, 193 pounds, and still growing is challenging. The baby industry is a licence to print money, too. Do you know how many hours I spent researching mattresses? Foam mattresses, organic mattresses, hard ones, soft ones, bio mattresses. My head was about to explode. I mean, what if I got it wrong? What if the one (or two) mattresses I bought were going to contain a deadly chemical that would be discovered in a few years to be associated with infant deaths? This made the basal-body-temperature-thermometer decision look like a piece of cake. Every decision was loaded with guilt, worry, and financial stress. My grandmother put her kids in a dresser drawer and here I was trying to source where the filling came from in an organic mattress! She would have laughed over her gin and tonic.

I was like a woman possessed in those final few weeks. But I have to say, thank God for Craigslist and those thoughtful women who post blogs on topics like "the complete list of things you do and do not need with twins." This saved both my sanity and my bank balance. Really, how did we manage before the internet?

I tend to be a last-minute person and childbirth was no exception. I was too late to sign up for prenatal classes, so at the same time that I was running around and trying to prepare, I was also madly trying to find a prenatal "crash course." About two weeks before the C-section date, I found a woman who would come to our house for several hours and give us the lowdown on giving birth and taking care of infants. Sam and I were very apprehensive about what she would tell us and she didn't disappoint. After a particularly detailed description of natural birth with twins, during which Sam slowly got paler and paler, she got out a twenty-four-hour clock. She then proceeded to tell us that we would have to feed the baby about every three hours.

Sounded reasonable until it became clear that, with two babies, the total feed time would take about two and a half hours. Sam quickly calculated that we would have about thirty minutes off before we had to start again.

"Good God, when do we sleep?" he asked.

"You don't," she replied. "But the good news for you is that it will be Julie doing most of the work if breastfeeding works out." I had stopped listening. I wanted her to put the twenty-four-hour clock away and go home. After she had gone, we were both very quiet.

"Don't worry," said Sam. "It will be fine. We'll manage."

I had already calculated that thirty minutes every three hours during a twenty-four-hour period was only two hundred and forty minutes—exactly four hours—of sleep maximum every twenty-four hours; not every eight hours, every twenty-four hours! This was not going to be fine.

At eight-and-a-half-months pregnant, I called Maxine. We had not spoken for a while since she had been dealing with the reality that carrying her own child might endanger her own life. I think she went quiet probably because of that news, but also no doubt because I was pregnant and she was still in the living hell of wanting, but not having, a child. After many conversations, Maxine and her husband had agreed that surrogacy was the answer. But deciding that was the way to go and actually doing it are two entirely different matters. Maxine had done some initial research and it was overwhelming. Not only would it cost probably close to $80,000, it was not even allowed in many states in the US.

When I called, I think Maxine was at a low point. "Why does it have to be so hard?" she said. "I've been through cancer and now I have to go through this crazy process to have a child. I just don't know if I have the energy."

This was probably the first time that I had heard her even come close to sounding like she was giving up on her dream.

"I just want someone to help me. The agency route is so expensive, but I'm not sure we have any other alternative."

"Well, I would donate my womb, Maxine." And I really meant it; I would have. "But it may need a while to recover after the birth of these two."

"No offence, but I don't rate your womb particularly well," she said. "It's not had a great track record. Plus you're thirty-nine. I think they prefer surrogates a good ten years younger."

"No offence taken. I probably wouldn't rate it well either! So what are you going to do?"

"I don't know," she said. "I'll figure it out." I felt sad when she put down the phone. Why was her journey so hard? We had both been firm believers that things happen for a reason and that we all have life lessons to learn. But, as Maxine said one day, "I must have been pretty bad-ass in a previous life to have to go through this in this one."

Maxine has never been one to feel sorry for herself for very long and I was not surprised when, about a week later, she called and let me know that she had decided not to go the agency route. She was going to campaign for a surrogate mother. She had written an email about her situation and had a list of close friends and relatives that she was going to send it to, asking whether they might know of anyone who would be willing to be a surrogate.

"Before you say anything," she said, "I know it's a complete bloody long shot, but I'm just putting it out to the universe. Maybe someone out there might want to help."

I couldn't help telling her that, although I thought it was a pretty gutsy thing to do, I wasn't sure it would garner much response. I had never heard of anyone saying yes to surrogacy via an email!

But I was wrong.

About a month later, Maxine called. She told me that her husband's second cousin had received the email, contacted them, and was willing to be the surrogate Mum! It was even more incredible, because she had already had three children: two boys and one girl. She felt she could handle another child of her own, but her husband had previously said no to a fourth child. On hearing Maxine's story, they had agreed that they wanted to help and that if everything worked out, Susan (the wife) could be the carrier.

"That is incredible, Max. What the hell!" I was so pleased for her. She said they had a long way to go and because Susan lived in a state where it was not allowed, there were a lot of challenges; but they were going to give it their best shot.

Over the next several months, Maxine's life was a round of lawyers, medical tests, clinic visits, flights, lawyers again, scans, remortgaging discussions, more tests, and stress. A lot of stress.

Finally, just before I was due to go in for my scheduled C-section, she phoned. They had defrosted six of her embryos and they were going to implant three. Susan had had a couple of medical issues, but had got the all clear and both were flying to the fertility clinic in Colorado the next morning for the transfer.

"This is it," she said. Five years after starting to try for a baby, she had a real shot at being a mother.

"How are you feeling?"

"Terrified," was her reply.

"Maxine, if anyone deserves this to work right now, it is you. I love you, Maxine."

She didn't call me after the transfer. I think, like me, she wanted to shut the world out until she knew the results. This was her one and only chance. There were no other options for her.

Eighteen days later, I got a call. "It worked," was all she said. "I'm finally going to be a Mum." We both burst into tears.

"The good news is, though," she said, "I still get to drink through my pregnancy."

This is why I love Maxine. She always has the last word.

The night before we were due to go in for the C-section, I was up painting pictures for the kids' room. The idea had seemed great at six months, but still not having completed it at thirty-eight-and-a-half weeks, I rather regretted trying to fit this in. At just after midnight, I finally finished. We had to get up at 5:00 a.m. the next morning to go to the hospital.

Sam and I didn't say much to each other that night. We knew

that the next day would be the start of a whole new life. What felt like the end of a journey was also the start. We were up at five, I put on my LUCKY pink t-shirt, which actually looked terrible now that it did not even fit over my belly, and we set off. I remember saying to Sam as we locked the door, "I think I would like them to stay inside; I'm not ready for when they come out!"

During the drive, I thought of our journey and of my friends' journeys. I think between all of us we had covered every possible way of having a child. Out of the seven of us, three had had children naturally, one through a sperm bank, one through adoption, one through IVF, and finally one through surrogacy. I think the only option left is the virgin birth and I knew none of us would qualify for that.

I also thought back on what the "dead" people had said. Remember the number "eight" which had made me book the second IVF for August? Well, the year I got pregnant was 2008, and I had conceived before the summer solstice, June 21st, as predicted by Gabrielle. I did not share this with Sam. He had endured enough.

We arrived at the hospital and the woman at reception said, "Well, by the size of you, I hope you are having twins." I have a good sense of humour, but at 5:30 in the morning, even my humour is a little thin.

It was a bit stressful going in for the epidural. The thought of the lower half of my body being paralyzed and staying awake for the procedure terrified me.

But walking into the operating theatre actually freaked me out more. I didn't realize that it would be so full of people. With twins, you have two sets of nurses, a pediatrician, my obstetrician, an anaesthetist, and I think someone else. It was like "theatre room rush hour" and it made me nervous. I lay down and chatted with the anaesthetist to take my mind off it. I really liked him, until I started dry retching as he fiddled with the anaesthetic to try and control the most excruciating headache.

Apart from this though, the operation went quite smoothly,

considering you have someone rummaging around in your abdomen trying to pull two new people out into this world.

I kept looking at Sam, because I knew his face would tell me if things were going okay and also to make sure he was still standing. The staff had been alerted that they had a "fainter" in the room—much to Sam's annoyance—but he stood firm. Even to the point—I found out later—that he took a picture of the placenta. Don't ask me why. I think through the IVF process, he had overcome some of his squeamishness and now he was feeling liberated. Placentas, umbilical cords, abdomen cut open—they are all in our "birth album."

Suddenly, the room went quiet. I could see on Sam's face that they were getting close to the birth. Despite being on lots of drugs, even I could tell that the tension in the room had increased. I remember closing my eyes and holding my breath. Please, please, let them be okay.

Then Baby A was out. It was 8:30 a.m. It was the boy. He was a bit blue, but okay.

By 8:35 a.m., Baby B, the girl was out. She was okay too.

They weighed in at six pounds and six-and-a-half pounds respectively. In case you forget to add, this is like carrying a twelve-and-a-half-pound baby, not counting the bits.

Sam held them first and told me they were perfect. It wasn't until that moment that I knew it had all been worth it. George and Francis Dexter had finally arrived.

To Summarize:

Years of trying: 5

Rounds of IVF: 3

Supplementary treatments: Every one you could possibly imagine and many more you probably can't.

Total $ spent: Best guess, $45,000 + (Have stopped counting.)

Sanity: You decide.

Relationship: A work in progress.

Epilogue

Sam and I

It has been five years since our twins were born. I honestly can't remember the first two years; they were a blur. I have never experienced exhaustion like that before. To the point where one day, when I had literally not slept for seventy-two hours, I bent down to do up my shoelace and stood up to see the stroller rolling through a gap between two parked cars and onto the main street. I was so spaced out, I couldn't figure out what was happening. Luckily, the chap next to me, who looked like he got a good eight hours every night, grabbed the stroller and saved my kids from potential disaster.

I was also back at work within five months, as we needed the money, so that came with a whole set of complications. Anyway, there are many stories about the last four years, but they are not for this book.

The two questions I get asked the most are: "Was it worth it?" and "How are you and Sam?"

Yes, of course, is the answer to the first, but there have been days when I really questioned both our decision to keep pursuing a child and our parenting abilities. But I know I am one of the lucky ones and I am grateful for that.

My response to the other question about, "How are you and Sam?" is, "You try having twins!" Let's just say our alcohol consumption has increased dramatically, but we are still together, trying to work it all out.

Maxine

At the time of writing, Maxine has just had her second baby through surrogacy. Her first son was born healthy about a year

169

after Francis and George arrived and now her family is complete with the arrival of her second son.

I have to hand it to her—she is one determined lady. Surrogacy is very stressful, complicated, and emotionally draining; and she persevered through it twice. I had to laugh as she recently visited us with her newborn and I expressed surprise at his being the most well-behaved child I have ever met. Her response was, "Well, I bloody hope so. He just cost me a second mortgage!" Seven years on, she remains cancer-free.

Debbie

Debs gave birth to a healthy son. Her relationship with her partner ended, but the good news is that the partner very much loves Debs' son and is still a big part of his life. Debs has relocated to a new place outside Vancouver and is in the process of setting up her new life. She would love another baby, but while juggling life as a single Mum, it is likely not going to happen—although with Debs you never know.

By the way, Chris (the friend who was going to be the original sperm donor) and his partner Ray are still very much together. No children of their own, but they are favourite uncles to Debs' little boy.

Kari

Kari's adopted twins from Vietnam are now five. She had a very tough few years too, but figured it out in the end. She is now building a new house and enjoying motherhood and the good life. In truth, I am a bit jealous of her lifestyle, but I'll get over it.

Jane and Mike

My sister and her husband are still going strong. Henry is an awesome little boy that my twins adore. I wish they lived closer as it would be good to see them more, and have a free babysitter, but we try and make it work as much as we can.

Lucy
Our super-fertile friend Lucy now has two children and has stopped at that. She is back at work after a strong realization that being a stay-at-home Mum was not for her. She is still passionate, Italian and loyal. If I were ever in any kind of fight—legal or otherwise—I would want her on my side.

Thalia
Thalia now has two beautiful boys and seems very happy in her marriage. She recently moved to a new part of town and is in the process of setting up a new business. We call Thalia and her husband "the happy couple." More of a reflection of our own issues rather than hers.

Caroline
I left Caroline till last. She has the briefest mention in this book, but is probably one of the main reasons for finally writing this story. As I finish this, Caroline, unlike Maxine who managed to beat cancer, is in the last days of her battle against the disease. At forty-four, she will be leaving behind a beautiful five-year-old boy, a beautiful three-year-old boy, and a loving husband. Her advice to me when I was telling her—not long after she was diagnosed with terminal cancer—that I was thinking about writing this was, "Well, get off your arse and get it done."
This one's for you, Caroline.
Thanks.

Author Biography

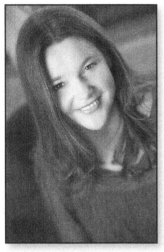

During Julie Selby's five-year infertility journey, she was told at one point that her chances of conceiving were less than ten percent even with medical intervention. To beat the odds, she tried everything to conceive from acupuncture, to immune testing, to trips to the psychic. Her insightful observations about the things she tried, the challenges she faced, and her determination to leave no stone unturned bring a humorous and refreshing approach to this highly emotional topic.

Today, Julie, a marketing and branding strategist, resides in Vancouver with her husband and is, very fortunately, the forty-five year old mother of five-year-old twins.

If you want to get on the path to be a published author with
Influence Publishing please go to
www.InfluencePublishing.com

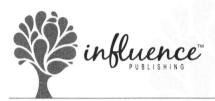

Inspiring books that influence change

More information on our other titles and how to submit your
own proposal can be found at
www.InfluencePublishing.com

.

Lightning Source UK Ltd.
Milton Keynes UK
UKOW06f1807190615

253798UK00014B/201/P